"THEY SAY IT'S 'JUST NERVES' . . ."

But it can stop you from working . . . upset your
personal relationships . . . transform you from the
busy and interesting person you used to be into
someone else. Dr. Claire Weekes has treated victims
of nervous illness with the care that only a sympathetic,
understanding doctor can offer. The man who has
trouble swallowing . . . the woman who cannot
travel outside the safety of her own home . . . the
young girl who is afraid she will be sick in public—
Dr. Weekes has answers for them all. She knows
about the tricks your nervous system can play on
you, and gives down-to-earth, step-by-step guidance
for achieving full recovery.

DR. CLAIRE WEEKES is the author of the bestselling
Peace from Nervous Suffering, also available in a
Signet edition. In addition, Dr. Weekes, best known
for her pioneering work in the study of nervous illness
and anxiety, has lectured at psychiatric hospitals
in Britain and has spoken often on radio and television
both in Britain and in the United States.

D0059317

Hope and Help
for Your Nerves

by
Dr. Claire Weekes,
M.B., D.Sc., M.R.A.C.P.

**Consulting Physician to the
Rachel Forster Hospital
Sydney, Australia**

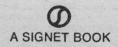

A SIGNET BOOK

SIGNET
Published by the Penguin Group
Penguin Books USA Inc., 375 Hudson Street,
New York, New York 10014, U.S.A.
Penguin Books Ltd, 27 Wrights Lane,
London W8 5TZ, England
Penguin Books Australia Ltd, Ringwood,
Victoria, Australia
Penguin Books Canada Ltd, 10 Alcorn Avenue,
Toronto, Ontario, Canada M4V 3B2
Penguin Books (N.Z.) Ltd, 182-190 Wairau Road,
Auckland 10, New Zealand

Penguin Books Ltd, Registered Offices:
Harmondsworth, Middlesex, England

Hope and Help for Your Nerves was previously published in a
Dutton edition.
First Signet Printing, September, 1990
11   10   9   8   7   6   5   4   3

 REGISTERED TRADEMARK—MARCA REGISTRADA

Printed in the United States of America

PUBLISHER'S NOTE
The ideas, procedures, and suggestions contained in this book are not intended as a
substitute for consulting with your physician. All matters regarding your health require
medical supervision.

To the memory of my indomitable mother

Many of those who suffer from nervousness are persons of fine susceptibilities and delicate regard for honor, endowed with a feeling of duty and obligation toward others. Their nerves have tricked them, misled them.

W. R. HOUSTON

Contents

Hope and Help for Your Nerves

1

The Power Within You

If you are reading this book because your nerves are "in a bad way," you are the very person for whom it has been written, and I shall therefore talk directly to you as if you were sitting beside me.

I shall show clearly and simply, and yet with all necessary detail, how such nervous illness begins and develops and how it can be cured. *The advice given here will definitely cure you, if you follow it*. This will take perseverance and some courage. You may notice that I have not asked for patience. A nervously ill person is rarely patient, because "sick" nerves are usually agitated nerves—that is one reason why he is bewildered by them. To wait patiently in line can be almost intolerable misery for such a person. However, there is a substitute for patience, and this I shall present to you later.

It will not be difficult for you to read this book: it is about you and your nerves, and for this reason you will read it with interest, whereas to read an ordinary book or newspaper may seem an impossibility or, should you succeed, may leave you more distressed than when you began.

I used the word "cure" and this may surprise you, because it implies an illness and you may think of yourself as more bewildered than ill, lost in a maze, trying to find your way back to being the person you used to be.

On the other hand, you may be so depressed and ex-

1

hausted that you may readily agree that you are ill. Whether or not you consider yourself ill, more than anything else you want to be yourself again. You probably look at others in the street and wonder why you can't be like them. What is this "terrible thing" that has happened to you? What is the meaning of these terrible feelings?

Such feelings may have possessed you for a long time, even for years. Indeed, you may have reached a point of such desperate suffering that you could be thinking of ending it all, or may even have attempted to do just that. And yet, however deeply involved you may be in nervous illness, however long you may have suffered, you can recover and enjoy life again. I emphasize *however deeply involved and however long*. The main difference between a person ill for many years and someone ill for a short time is that the one who suffered for long has had more time to collect disturbing memories, especially the memory of much defeat, so that he despairs easily. But there is nothing altered within this person determining that because he has been ill for so long, he cannot possibly recover now.

However long you may have been ill, your body is waiting to recover in exactly the same way as the body of a person who has been ill for only a short time. It is important to understand this, because your illness is very much an illness of how you think. It is very much an illness of your attitude to fear, panic. You may think it is an illness of how you feel (it most certainly seems like this), but how you feel depends on how you think, on what you think. Because it is an illness of what you think, you can recover. *Thoughts that are keeping you ill can be changed*. In other words, your approach to your illness can be changed.

Now don't despair when you read this. I know how easily you despair and how impossible it may seem to you at this moment to imagine changing your approach to your illness. It is my work to show you how to do this, to help you do this. Have the courage to read on and see what you must do. Don't despair. Take heart!

When I see a person who has suffered from nervous illness for a long while, I do not think of him or her as hopelessly, chronically ill. Neither do I see a coward. I see a suffering, bewildered person, who has possibly not had adequate explanation of his illness, adequate help. So many people have been cured at last after having been ill for many years that no one should be discouraged by a history of long illness.

The guidance you need is in this small book. The perseverance you can, with help, find within yourself. *The strength to recover is within you, once you are shown the way.* I assure you of this.

Each of us has unsuspected power to accomplish what we demand of ourselves, if we care to search for it. You are no exception. You can find it if you make up your mind to, however great a coward you may think yourself at this moment. I have no illusions about you: I am not writing this book for the rare brave people, but for you, a sick, suffering, ordinary human being with no more courage than the rest of us but—and this is the important thing—with the same unplumbed, unsuspected power in reserve as the rest of us. It is possible that you may be aware of such power but may feel, because of your nervous condition, unable to release it. This book will help you find this power, and show you how to use it.

First, you must know how your nervous system works.

2

How Our Nervous System Works

Our nervous system consists of two main parts, known as voluntary and involuntary (autonomic).

THE VOLUNTARY NERVES

These nerves direct the movement of limbs, head, and trunk, and we control them more or less as we wish, hence their name, voluntary. They consist of brain and spinal cord, from which a number of paired nerves arise, each ending in the muscle it supplies.

THE INVOLUNTARY NERVES

Endocrine glands govern and regulate the normal functions of our body, including our body's reaction to stress. They do this with the help of involuntary nerves that act as their messengers. The involuntary nerves have their headquarters in a brain center connected with a delicate network of fibers (involuntary nerves) lying on either side of the spinal column (backbone), from which numerous threadlike branches pass to the internal organs—heart, lungs, intestines, etc. Unlike the voluntary nerves, the involuntary nerves are not under our direct control but—and this is of paramount importance in understanding "nerves"—*they respond to our moods*. For example, when we are afraid, our cheeks blanch, our pupils dilate, our heart races, and our hands may sweat. We do not consciously react this way and we have no power to stop these reactions *other than to change our mood.* This is why we call these nerves involuntary.

The involuntary nerves themselves consist of two parts, the sympathetic and the parasympathetic. Of these, the sympathetic "sympathizes" more demonstratively with our moods, hence its name. The action of the sympathetic nerves strengthens an animal's defenses against the various dangers that beset it, such as extremes of temperature, deprivation of water, attack by its enemies, *any form of stress.*

Have you ever seen a frightened animal standing stock-still from fear before taking flight? Its nostrils and its pupils dilate, its heart races, it breathes quickly. The sympathetic nerves, taking signal from the endocrine glands and acting as their messengers, have prepared the animal for fight or flight.

THE PATTERN OF FEAR

We human beings react in the same way when afraid. Fear begins as an impulse in our brain that excites the sympathetic nerves to stimulate various regions (skin) and organs (heart, lungs, eyes) to produce the signs and symptoms of fear—the sweating hands, racing heart, quick breathing, dry mouth, etc. The sympathetic nerves do this mainly by a chemical called adrenalin, which is released at the nerve terminals in the organs concerned. Also, our two adrenal glands, themselves under sympathetic nervous stimulation, secrete additional adrenalin into our bloodstream to enhance the action of the sympathetic nerves.

When we are afraid we also feel a horrible sensation in the "pit of the stomach." This is the most distressing component of fear. However, the complete picture of fear includes all the symptoms induced by adrenalin: the sweating hands, churning stomach, racing heart, tight chest, etc., as well as the spasm of fear left in our "middle."

Normally we do not feel our body functioning, because parasympathetic nerves hold the sympathetic nerves in check. It is only when we are overwrought (angry, afraid, excited) that the sympathetic nerves dominate the parasympathetic and we are conscious of certain organs functioning. A healthy body without stress is a peaceful body.

Most of us associate kindness and understanding with the word "sympathetic," and as the reactions of the sympathetic nerves can be anything but kind, some people find it difficult to reconcile themselves to the term "sympathetic nerves." Therefore, to avoid bewilderment, I shall henceforth refer to the sympathetic nerves as the adrenalin-releasing nerves. Adrenalin is not the only hormone concerned with expressing emotion, particularly stress. However, for the sake of simplicity, I am concerned only with it.

So, briefly, we have voluntary nerves by means of which we move our body; and involuntary nerves consisting of adrenalin-releasing nerves and parasympathetic divisions that help to control the functions of our internal organs, each part checking the other. Normally we do not feel our involuntary nerves working, but when we are overwrought, the adrenalin-releasing nerves are especially stimulated and we may feel our heart beat quickly, our hands may sweat, and our mouth feel dry. In addition, our stomach may "churn," we may feel breathless, giddy, and may have an urgent need to retire to the toilet.

3

What Is Nervous Breakdown?

It will be appreciated that there are different grades of "nervous" suffering. Countless people have "bad nerves" and many of them, although distressed, continue at their work and cannot be said to suffer from nervous breakdown. Indeed, while they readily admit to having "bad nerves" they would indignantly refute any suggestion of breakdown. And yet a nervous breakdown is no more than an intensification of their symptoms. Although this book is concerned mainly with the development and treatment of nervous breakdown, almost every symptom complained of by people with "bad nerves" will be found here, and such people will recognize themselves again and again in the patients with breakdown described in the following pages. *The symptoms are the same, it is but their severity that varies.* The person with breakdown feels these symptoms much more intensely.

Where do "bad nerves" end and where does nervous breakdown begin? By nervous breakdown we mean a state in which a person's "nervous" symptoms are so intense that he copes inadequately with his daily work or does not cope at all. To put it more scientifically and more fully, by nervous breakdown we mean a major interruption in the body's efficient functioning as a result of emotional and mental fatigue brought on and maintained by stress, mainly by fear.

The term "nervous breakdown" has an ominous sound to the average person and is veiled in mystery and confusion. Doctors are asked if people really "break," and if so, how? We are also asked how a nervous breakdown begins and what causes it.

THE BREAKING POINT

Many people are tricked into breakdown. A continuous state of fear, whatever the cause, gradually stimulates the adrenalin-releasing nerves to produce *a set pattern* of disturbing sensations. These are well known to doctors but so little known to people generally that, when first experienced, they may bewilder and dupe their victims into becoming afraid of them. If asked to pinpoint the beginning of a nervous breakdown, I would say that it is at this moment when the sufferer becomes *afraid* of the alarming, strange sensations produced by continuous fear and tension and so places himself, or herself, in the circle of fear-adrenalin-fear. *This is the breaking point.* In response to growing fear, more and more adrenalin is released and organs are stimulated to produce even more intense sensations, which inspire still more fear. The circle goes around and around until the sufferer becomes lost and confused.

TWO TYPES OF BREAKDOWN

Most nervously ill people who have come to me for help have had either one of two different types of breakdown. The first is relatively straightforward, and its victim is mainly concerned with physical symptoms, disturbing sensations, *the way he feels*. This person has minor problems only, such as an inability, because of illness, to cope with his responsibilities. We call this kind of illness an Anxiety State, and it is the simplest form of Anxiety State we know.

The second type of breakdown is begun by some overwhelming problem, sorrow, guilt, or disgrace. Continuous tension and prolonged, anxious brooding arising from these causes may not only eventually produce the physical symptoms of stress found in the first type of breakdown but may also bring certain distressing experiences, such as indecision, suggestibility, loss of confidence, feelings of unreality, feelings of personality disintegration, obsession, depression. The sufferer may finally become just as concerned with these sensations, these experiences, as with the original cause of his illness; indeed, he may become more concerned with them. This, too, is an Anxiety State but more complicated than the first one described above.

In this book I am concerned only with these two types—the most usual types—of breakdown. The term "breakdown" is unscientific and unnecessarily alarming, and the term "Anxiety State" is too "medical" for the purpose of this book, so I will henceforth avoid using them where possible and will replace them with the term "nervous illness."

4

The Commonest, Simplest Form of Nervous Illness

People suffering from the commonest, simplest form of nervous illness (simplest form of Anxiety State) complain of some, or all, of the following symptoms: fatigue, churning stomach, indigestion, racing heart, banging heart, palpitations, "missed" heartbeats, a sharp pain under the heart, a sore feeling around the heart, sweating hands, "pins and needles" in the hands and feet (especially the hands), a choking feeling in the throat, an inability to take in a deep breath, a tight feeling across the chest, "ants" crawling under the skin, a tight band of pain around the head, a heavy weight pressing on top of the head, giddiness, strange tricks of vision such as the apparent movement of inanimate objects, weak "spells," sleeplessness, depression. Nausea, occasional vomiting, diarrhea, and the frequent desire to pass urine may be added to the list.

The following is a typical list brought to the doctor by such a patient. This was brought by a young mother. It is printed exactly as she wrote it:

All tied up
Headaches
Tired and weary
Palpitations
Dreadful

Nervous
Sharp pain under the heart
No interest
Restless
My heart beats like lead
I have a heavy lump of dough in my stomach
Heart shakes

Sufferers from these symptoms are quite certain that there is something seriously wrong with them and cannot believe that anyone else could have had such a distressing experience. Many feel convinced that they have a brain tumor (at least something "deep seated") or that they are on the verge of insanity. Their one wish is to be, as quickly as possible, the person they used to be before this "horrible thing" happened to them. They are rarely aware that their symptoms are nervous (emotional) in origin and follow a well-recognized pattern shared by numerous sufferers like themselves, *the pattern of continuous fear and tension.*

THE THREE MAIN PITFALLS
LEADING INTO NERVOUS ILLNESS

Three main pitfalls can lead into nervous illness. They are *sensitization, bewilderment, and fear.* Sensitization is a state in which our nerves react in an exaggerated way to stress; that is, they bring very intense feelings when under stress and they may react this way with alarming swiftness, almost in a flash. There is no mystery about sensitization. We have all surely felt it in a mild way at the end of a day's tense work, when our nerves feel on edge and little things upset us too much. Constant tension alerts nerves to react in a mildly exaggerated way. It's not pleasant and we don't like it. If it is more severe, we may be alarmed and think that our nerves are in a very bad way indeed. *So much nervous illness is no more than severe sensitization kept alive by bewilderment and fear.*

The Cleaner's Broom Against His Bed

Severe sensitization can come suddenly or gradually. It can come suddenly following a shock to our nervous system, such as an exhausting surgical operation, a severe hemorrhage, a difficult confinement, an accident. For example, a patient "without a nerve in his body" may go to the hospital for an operation and after the operation may awaken to find that the gentle impact of a cleaner's broom against his bed may shoot through him like a whipping flash and the strain of waiting for visitors to arrive may bring such agitation that waiting may seem intolerable. Severe sensitization may come more gradually following too strenuous dieting; severe anemia; indeed following any debilitating illness; or it may accompany the constant tension of being in some difficult life situation such as living with an alcoholic husband or wife, an incompatible in-law, an erring child. In other words, long, anxious brooding on *any* difficult life situation may gradually bring sensitization.

At the End of the Pew
At the Back of the Church

Also, some nervously ill people have no cause for their illness as apparent as those just mentioned, and much time may then be spent searching in such people for deep-seated causes—so called subconscious causes —in the hope that by finding them the patient may be cured. While exposing a hidden cause for nervous illness may be interesting, I have rarely seen it help a person who has been ill for a long time. *Present sensitization remains to be cured,* whatever the original cause. The sensitized person is concerned with *the state he is in now,* not with what may possibly have caused it a long time ago. He is afraid of so much. On Sunday he sits at the end of the pew at the back of the church, so that he can slip outside unnoticed if, as he thinks, his fears grow beyond him. At the school function, at the restaurant, he sits near the door, "Just in case, just in case!"

When a person is constantly sensitized and afraid of the state he is in, we say he is nervously ill. Fear must come into the picture to bring this kind of illness. Sensitization alone is not enough, because without fear a body will quickly repair its sensitized state.

The Simple Shock
of Tripping in the Dark

The feeling of fear that a sensitized person experiences can be very intense. The simple shock of tripping in the dark may be enough to bring a flash of panic to a severely sensitized person. Also, under the constant strain of anxiety about the way he feels, such a person may find that, from time to time, he may feel all the upsetting symptoms I described above—the churning stomach, racing heart, sweating hands, etc.

They Fear the Unknown
As Much As the Known

As I have already mentioned, very few nervously ill people realize that their symptoms follow a well-known pattern shared by numerous sufferers like themselves, the pattern of continuous fear and tension. They do not understand that theirs are the normal symptoms of stress, the ordinary symptoms of anxiety, made intense by sensitization. They do not know that their symptoms are caused by adrenalin secreted when they are afraid, anxious. Nor do they know that adrenalin can act only on certain organs and then only in a certain way and that this is why the pattern of their symptoms is set, limited. The pattern is so set that many nervously ill people have already experienced the worst their nerves can bring them, but they do not know this. Their body has brought so many frightening surprises in the past that they live in constant fear of what further surprise may yet be in store. They fear the unknown as much as they fear the known. They may fear the unknown more than the known, so they live anxiously, tensely wondering what will happen next. Their very anxiety determines that symptoms will

continue to come, but whatever new symptoms may
arise, they are always part of the same pattern of stress,
still part of an expected pattern.

CONCERNED WITH THE WAY THEY FEEL

I wish to stress very strongly that many sufferers
from nervous illness have no specific problem keeping
them ill, other than finding the way to recovery. *The
great majority of my nervously ill patients have been
made ill and kept ill because of the way they feel;
because of fear of what they think may happen next.*

I will now describe, step by step, the development
and cure of such an illness, and you may recognize
much of yourself in the person described here.

THE BEGINNING: PALPITATIONS

Many people, sensitized by one of the many causes
described above, are precipitated into nervous illness by
the fear induced by some sudden, alarming, yet harmless bodily sensation such as their first unexpected attack of palpitations. Such an attack can be frightening
to a highly strung temperament, especially if it comes
at night and there is no one to turn to for comfort and
reassurance. The heart races wildly and the sufferer is
sure it will burst. He usually lies still, afraid to move
for fear of further damaging himself. *So fear arises.*
It is only natural to be alarmed by sudden, unexpected,
uncomfortable happenings in our body, particularly in
the region of our heart.

FEAR-ADRENALIN-FEAR CYCLE

Fear causes an additional outpouring of adrenalin,
so that a heart already stirred to palpitations becomes
further excited, beats even more quickly, and the attack lasts longer. The sufferer may panic, thinking he
is about to die. His hands sweat, his face burns, his
fingers tingle with "pins and needles" while he waits
for he knows not what.

The attack eventually stops—it always does—and all may be well for a while. However, having had one frightening experience, he dreads another and for days remains tense and anxious, from time to time feeling his pulse. If the palpitations do not return he settles down, loses himself in his work and forgets the incident. If, however, he has a second attack, he really is concerned. Apparently the wretched thing has come to stay!

Not only is he afraid of palpitating, but he is also in a state of tension, wondering what further alarming experience may yet be in store for him. It is not long before tension, releasing more and more adrenalin, makes his stomach churn, his hands sweat, and his heart constantly beat quickly. He becomes even more afraid, and still more adrenalin is released. In other words, he becomes caught in the fear-adrenalin-fear cycle.

TENSION THROUGH FEAR. "DON'T OVERDO IT!"

At this stage the sufferer consults a doctor, who usually succeeds in reassuring him and banishing his fear. However, he may not be sufficiently reassured and may be unfortunate enough to be put to bed and advised to "Take things carefully" and to "Be sure not to overdo it." When so advised, the average person, particularly if young and not yet protected by the philosophy of age, lies in bed brooding over his "bad" heart, afraid to move for fear of straining it further. This patient was already in a state of nervous tension worrying about the palpitations. Can you imagine his tension now? Perhaps you have experienced it.

On the other hand, should the doctor, in an effort to reassure him, make too light of the palpitations, the patient may stay in bed of his own volition, convinced that the doctor is withholding the worst and has not told him all. If he remains tense and afraid, he is certain to have further attacks, and the more frequently they come the more he hugs the couch. The more he rests, the more time he has to brood and the more tense and apprehensive he becomes. His finger is constantly hovering above his pulse, and in response to this anxiety his heart constantly beats more quickly than it should, although not so fast as when palpitating. Actually he thinks it is beating faster than it is, because he is conscious of every beat. To him it is thumping, banging, racing. One ingenious woman arranged her pillows end to end, so that she could lay her ear on the crack between them. In this way she thought she heard less thumping.

The sufferer by now is really sorry for himself. He loses appetite, loses weight, and dreads being alone "for fear of having a spell"; at the same time he is afraid to be with people for fear of having one and making a fool of himself. It is not long before he develops most of the sensations of nervous illness—the churning stomach, giddiness, headache, pains around the heart, etc.—in other words, the full fear-adrenalin-fear cycle.

FEAR OF SOME OTHER UPSETTING BODILY SENSATION

If fear of palpitations has not drawn this person into this type of illness, fear of some other upsetting bodily sensation generally has. Perhaps he has had pain in the region of his heart that he, in alarm and ignorance, diagnoses as angina. Perhaps a strenuous, highly tensed life has given him a constantly churning stomach or "shaking" heart at which he becomes alarmed. Whatever the cause, in answer to his continuous apprehension his adrenalin-releasing nerves become sensitized, always ready to trigger off the upsetting sensations described above. He tries to fight or escape, until he, too, becomes caught in the same fear-adrenalin-fear cycle as the person afraid of the palpitations.

As mentioned, nervously ill people have these sensations as a more or less constant background to their day. They may have moments of respite; for example, some on waking feel strangely calm and may be able to lie at peace for an hour or so before the churning starts. Others feel calmest at night. Others know no peace.

PANIC

Some people, as well as having this background of disturbing sensations, are swept from time to time by intense waves of panic. It will be appreciated how disturbing this panic can be when a sufferer is working and trying to appear normal and how he lives in dread of its coming at inappropriate moments. Unfortunately it is most likely to come at such times, as he is then most apprehensive and afraid.

It is possible that the recurring attacks of palpitation have now left him and that he is more concerned with the other manifestations of fear, although it is more usual to find the palpitations continuing and adding to the miserable burden.

"WHY DOESN'T HE PULL UP HIS SOCKS?"

This is not a far-fetched story. I have heard it so often that I give it respectful attention. I have known this stage, inadequately treated, to last years, the patient going from doctor to doctor.

To healthy people this history may sound all too childish and stupid. They think, "Why doesn't he pull up his socks and get on with his work and forget all this nonsense?" That is exactly what he would like to do. But what we, the healthy ones, do not realize is that by this time the fear felt by such a sufferer is greater than any the average person has known or has paused to imagine. Repeated spasms of panic, when accompanied by exhaustion and sensitization, not only increase in intensity but need less and less to start them. Dread of having them may bring on a whole sequence. Meeting a stranger, the thought of being left alone, even a slamming door may suffice. Also, in spite of a great desire to pull up his socks and get to work, such frequent, intense spasms of fear seem to paralyze his will to act.

Some years ago, when recuperating from an operation, I stayed with friends who were planning a hike. They asked a young man to join us. It was not a long walk, they assured me (but long enough for me, thought I, as I looked at his long legs). To my astonishment this big fellow soon fell behind and we frequently had to wait for him to catch up. At lunch he lay exhausted on the grass. Later he told me his story. For years, since student days, he had had recurring spasms of intense panic, so that his life had become a nightmare. He was not afraid of anything in particular, only of the feeling of fear itself, and this had become so intense and exhausting that even that short walk had seemed too much.

This man was eventually cured with explanation and was able to lead a scientific expedition. I mention him because he was no weakling but a clever scientist in a responsible position. He recovered quickly with help, after having suffered for ten years.

FIGHTING

The sufferer from nervous illness is neither fool nor coward, but often a remarkably brave person who fights his breakdown to the best of his ability with commendable although often misdirected courage. He may fight through almost every waking moment, with sweating hands and tensed muscles, agitatedly trying to force forgetfulness of his desperate state by consciously forcing concentration on other things. Or he may pace the floor of his mind, anxiously searching for a way out of his miserable prison, only to meet one closed door after another.

At night he falls into bed exhausted, to sleep the fretful sleep of nervous agitation, the heavy sleep of nervous exhaustion, the drugged sleep of the barbiturate swallower, or, worse still, to find no sleep in spite of heavy sedation.

At times the early evening may not seem so bad.

He may feel almost normal and think he has conquered this "thing" at last, and may go to bed saying, "Now, that's the finish. Tomorrow I will be my old self again," only to wake and find the spasms and churning as severe as ever. He cannot understand why, having felt so much better by evening, he should wake the next morning feeling as ill as ever, perhaps even worse. He certainly feels more hopeless, if that is possible. He is either convinced that there is some short road to recovery that continually eludes him, or that there is not, and never could be, a way back to peace from such suffering as his.

"YOU'LL HAVE TO
FIGHT THIS THING, OLD MAN!"

He looks back with longing at the person he used to be, the person who could sit peacefully and enjoy a good book, or happily watch television, and he apprehensively counts the weeks, months, years since he was that person. He reasons that if he cannot become himself again by fighting, how else can he? Fighting is his natural defense, the only weapon he knows, so he fights even harder. *But the harder he fights, the worse he becomes.* Naturally—*fighting means more tension, tension more adrenalin and further stimulation of the adrenalin-releasing nerves, and so the continuation of symptoms.* To make matters worse, his friends do not hesitate to advise him to fight it. Even his doctor may say, "You'll have to fight this thing, old man. You mustn't let it get the better of you!"

What has happened to him he cannot understand. He is like a man possessed. He does not realize that there is no devil sitting on his shoulder and that he is simply *doing this to himself with fear, fight, and flight from fear.*

It is at this stage that he may develop severe headache, which he likens to an iron band encircling his head, or to a weight pressing on top of it. He may be giddy, nauseated, have difficulty in expanding his chest to take in a deep breath, feel a heavy soreness around his heart or a sharp pain under it, which he sometimes refers to as "the dagger." He may also have recurring "funny spells" such as attacks of weakness, "missed" heartbeats, trembling turns, and spells of abnormally slowly beating heart. He loses interest in everything and in everybody, and mounting tension makes him easily upset by trifles. As one young mother put it, "I take it out on the poor kids."

SEDATION

The doctor usually prescribes sedatives at this stage, and there is no doubt that the patient may need them. But with a layman's distrust of such "dope," his family is probably urging him to "Throw the wretched stuff down the sink," adding, "It is only helping to depress you," and "That doctor will make an addict out of you if you don't watch out!" The sufferer becomes further confused because at the back of his mind he, too, is afraid of that. Part of a doctor's problem is to convince the patient—and, what is just as important, the patient's family—that such sedation is not only *not* harmful but, as a temporary measure, may be very necessary, and that it will not make an addict of him if carefully supervised. Usually when cured, the last thing these people want to see is one of those wretched capsules or a dose of that pink mixture.

Life is so contrary, it can put many unexpected obstacles in the way of recovery. In the words of one woman, "You would never believe the numbers of monkey wrenches that get thrown into the works."

For example, it is possible that, just as the doctor is winning the battle over taking sedatives, someone chooses that moment to take an overdose of barbiturates and the newspapers will be vociferous on the dangers of taking such drugs. The patient, who probably hasn't looked at a paper for weeks, somehow never fails to see that report or hear about it, and so the doctor's battle begins again.

And yet, however sedated this person may be, fear usually finds its way through such sedation. Sedation only softens the blow, but it does do that, and so plays an important part in recovery, as will be discussed later.

"DOCTOR, HE HAS COLLAPSED!"

Finally the day may come when, yielding to some extra burden of fear, the sufferer gives up what he thinks is his last ounce of strength and "collapses," while the alarmed family stands around helplessly. The words heard murmured in the hall, "Doctor, he has collapsed!" close a chapter for him and act as chains to bind him to the bed. If he could not find his way out of his illness while on his two feet, he wonders how he will find it now that he has collapsed. The fight seems too great, the journey too uphill, so he may spend weeks, even months, on his back, or be taken to a hospital for special treatment.

THE CONSTANT PATTERN OF FEAR

No doubt you have recognized some of yourself in this person, and it may be a revelation to find that the basis of your mysterious symptoms is, like his, fear.

Whether breakdown be mild or severe, *the basic cause is fear*. Conflict, problems, sorrow, guilt, or disgrace may start a breakdown, but it is not long before fear takes command. Even great sorrow at the loss of a loved one is mixed with fear, the fear of facing the future alone. Sexual problems are most likely to cause breakdown when accompanied by fear or guilt. Guilt opens the door to fear. Anxiety, worry, dread are only variants of fear in different guises.

ADA HAS MIGRAINE

It could be argued that strain, as distinct from fear, may cause breakdown in certain situations. For example, there is much prolonged strain for a middle-aged woman tending an old, sick parent. However, while she copes from day to day, does not look too far ahead, and does not think it too important that she is literally chained to her duties, she can sustain months, years of such strain. She may "bend" and need help from time to time, but she will not "break."

I once commented on the ability of one woman to carry on for so long in such a situation and was told by her brother, "Yes, it is a great strain on Ada, but Ada never did think of herself." That was the key to Ada's endurance. Had Ada listened to her sympathizing friends, begun to feel sorry for herself, and come to dread the future, she would have sown the seeds of nervous illness.

Strain may cause severe headache (Ada had migraine) and physical exhaustion, but unless accompanied by constant fear it will not cause the incapacity known as nervous illness. When work threatens to become beyond our physical strength and our responsibilities demand that we keep going, fear usually comes into the picture, and any ensuing nervous illness is caused not by the exhaustion, as so many believe, but by the fears it brings.

AFRAID TO ADMIT FEAR

Sometimes it is difficult for a person to admit even to himself that he is afraid. One woman insisted that it was the "stomach shakes," not fear, that caused her nervousness. So I avoided the word "fear" when talking to her and substituted the word "tension." Her stomach had "shaken" for six months; she had eaten little, slept little, and looked the wreck she felt, and yet when she finally accepted that the shakes depended on the excretion of adrenalin through tension, she was able to relax and lose them within a month. However, she continued to insist that she had not been afraid of them.

Is it possible to explain the disappearance of this woman's symptoms in any other way than that she had lost her fear of them? I asked her for an explanation and she said "I disliked them. I lost my dislike of them." She had disliked them so much that she had let them dominate her life for six months. Surely the difference between such strong dislike and fear is only one of degree? At least we have to admit that strong dislike of physical sensation is so close to fear that it can cause the same nervous reactions.

Camouflage your fear as intense dislike if it makes you feel happier. This is not important, as long as you understand that the physical reactions in your body to intense dislike and fear are so similar that any difference between them is negligible.

THE SINGLE PATTERN

The nervous illness described in this chapter was not complicated by a particular problem. It was caused by no more than *fear of the very feelings that fear itself had aroused,* and as such is the commonest and most straightforward form of nervous illness we know. If yours is this type of illness, it is a step toward cure to see your various symptoms as part of a single pattern coming from a single cause, fear. *These symptoms are not peculiar to you, but are well known to many like you.*

However distressing your symptoms may be, I assure you that every unwelcome sensation can be banished and you can regain peace of mind and body.

5

Cure of the Commonest Kind of Nervous Illness

If you have the kind of nervous illness just described, you will notice that, as already mentioned, you have certain symptoms as a fairly constant background to your day, while others come from time to time. For example, the churning stomach, sweating hands, and rapidly beating heart may be more or less always with you; while fear spasms, palpitations, "missed" heartbeats, pains around the heart, trembling spells, breathlessness, giddiness, nausea come in attacks at intervals. The constant symptoms are those of sustained tension and fear, hence their chronicity; while the different recurring attacks are the result of varying intensity in sustained fear, hence their periodicity.

"This Is Too Simple for Me"

The treatment of all symptoms depends on a few simple rules. When you first read them you may think, "This is too simple for me. It will take something more drastic to cure me." In spite of this, you will need to be shown how to apply this simple treatment and may often have to reread instructions.

The principle of treatment can be summarized as:

Facing
Accepting

Floating
Letting time pass

There is nothing mysterious or surprising about this treatment, and yet it is enlightening to see how many people sink deeper into their illness by *doing the exact opposite*.

Let us look again briefly at the person described in the last chapter, the person afraid of the physical feelings aroused by fear, and see if we can pinpoint his own treatment of his illness.

First, he became unduly alarmed by his symptoms, examining each as it appeared, "listening in" in apprehension. He tried to free himself of the unwelcome feelings by tensing himself to meet them or by pushing them away, agitatedly seeking occupation to force forgetfulness—in other words, by fighting or running away.

Also, he was bewildered because he could not find cure overnight. He kept looking back and worrying because so much time was passing and he was not yet cured, as if this were an evil spirit that could be exorcised if only he, or the doctor, knew the trick. *He was impatient with time*.

Briefly, he spent his time:

Running away, not facing;
Fighting, not accepting;
Arresting and "listening in," not floating past;
Being impatient with time, not letting time pass.

Need we be impressed if he thinks it will take something more drastic than facing, accepting, floating, and letting time pass to cure him? I don't think we need.

Now, let us consider how you can cure yourself by *facing, accepting, floating, and letting time pass*.

We will first consider cure of the constant symptoms and then of the recurring attacks.

6

Cure of the More Constant Symptoms

First, look at yourself and notice how you are sitting in your chair. I have no doubt that you are tensely shrinking from the feelings within you and yet, at the same time, are ready to "listen in" in apprehension. I want you to do *the exact opposite*. I want you to sit as comfortably as you can, relax to the best of your ability by letting your arms and legs sag into the chair as if charged with lead. In other words, let your body "flop" in the chair. Now examine and *do not shrink from* the sensations that have been upsetting you. I want you to examine each carefully, *to analyze and describe it aloud to yourself*. For example, you may say, "My hands sweat and tremble. They feel sore. . . ." This may sound a little silly and you may smile. So much the better.

CHURNING STOMACH

Begin with the nervous feeling in your stomach, the so-called churning. This may feel like an uneasy fluttering or may bore steadily like a hot poker passing from your stomach to your back. Do not tensely flinch from it. Go with it. Relax and analyze it. Take a few minutes to do this before reading on.

Now that you have faced and examined it, is it so

terrible? If you had arthritis in your wrist, you would be prepared to work with the arthritic pain without becoming too upset. Why regard this churning as something so different from ordinary pain that it can frighten you? Stop regarding it as some monster trying to possess you. Understand that it is but the working of oversensitized adrenalin-releasing nerves and that by constantly shrinking from it you have stimulated an excessive outflow of adrenalin that has further excited your nerves to produce continual churning. *By your anxiety you are producing the very feelings you dislike so much.*

While you examine and analyze this churning a strange thing may happen: you may find your attention wandering from yourself. This "thing," which seemed so terrible while you stayed tense and flinched from it, may fail to hold your attention for long when you see it for what it is—no more than a strange physical feeling of no great medical significance, and causing no real harm.

Just As a Broken Leg Takes Time to Heal

So, *be prepared to accept and live with it for the time being.* Accept it as something that will be with you for some time yet—in fact while you recover—but something that will eventually leave you if you are prepared to let time pass and not anxiously watch the churning during its passing.

But do not make the mistake of thinking that it will go *as soon as you cease to fear it.* Your nerves are still sensitized and will take time to heal, just as a broken leg takes time. However, as you improve and are no longer afraid of the churning, and do not try to cure it by controlling it, and are prepared to accept it and work with it present, you will gradually become more interested in other things and will gradually forget to notice whether it is there or not. *This is the way to recover.* By true acceptance you break the fear-adrenalin-fear cycle or, in other words, the churning-adrenalin-churning cycle.

TRUE ACCEPTANCE:
THE KEYSTONE TO RECOVERY

From this discussion you will appreciate that true acceptance is the keystone to recovery, and before you continue with the examination of your other symptoms we should make sure that you understand its exact meaning.

I find that some patients complain, "I have accepted that churning in my stomach, but it is still there. So what am I to do now?" How could they have accepted it while they still complain about it?

Or, as one old man said, "After breakfast the churning starts. I can't just sit there and churn. If I do, I'm exhausted after an hour, so I have to get up and walk around. But I'm too tired to walk around, so what am I to do?" I said to him, "You haven't really accepted that churning, have you?" "Oh yes, I have," he answered indignantly. "I'm not frightened of it any more."

But he obviously was. He was afraid that after an hour's churning he would be exhausted, so he sat tensely dreading its arrival, shrinking from it when it came and worrying about the exhaustion to follow. Of course the churning, itself a symptom of tension, *must inevitably come while so tensely awaited.*

I tried to make him understand that he must be prepared to let his stomach churn and to continue reading his paper *while it churned.* He must try to loosen that tight hold on himself, literally let his body sag into the chair and go toward, not shrink from, any feeling his body brings him. Only by so doing would he be truly accepting. In this way, and only in this way, would he eventually reach the stage when it would no longer matter whether his stomach churned or not. Then, freed from the stimulus of tension and anxiety, his adrenalin-releasing nerves would gradually calm down and the churning would automatically lessen and finally cease.

THE SYMPTOMS ARE ALWAYS A REFLECTION OF YOUR MOOD

This man was asked to do no more than change his mood from apprehension to acceptance. *The symptoms of this type of illness are always a reflection of your mood.* However, it is well to remember that it may be some time before your body reacts to the new mood of acceptance and that it may continue for a while to reflect the tense, frightened mood of the preceding weeks, months, or years. This is one reason why nervous illness can be so bewildering and why this old man was bewildered. He had begun to accept, but when the symptoms did not disappear immediately, he quickly lost heart and became apprehensive again, although trying to convince himself that he was accepting. *It takes time for a body to establish acceptance as a mood and for this eventually to bring peace,* just as it took time for fear to become established as continuous tension and anxiety. That is why "letting time pass" is such an important part of your treatment and why I emphasize it again and again. Time is the answer. *But there must be that background of true acceptance while waiting for time to pass.*

SWEATING, TREMBLING HANDS

Now look at your hands. They sweat? They tremble? Maybe the skin is sore and tingles with "pins and needles"? But the hands of any frightened, tense person may feel like that and you are certainly frightened, so how could your hands behave otherwise? The sweating, trembling, "pins and needles," and soreness are no more than the physical expression of *oversensitization of your adrenalin-releasing nerves through anxiety and fear*. These sensations get no worse than this and could never prevent your using your hands. Maybe your hands do sweat and tremble, but *they are still good hands to use*.

Therefore, accept the sweating, trembling, soreness, and tingling *for the time being*. These cannot be cured overnight. With acceptance, although your hands may still tremble and sweat for a while, you will find some peace, enough to begin to still the outflow of adrenalin so that your sweat glands will gradually calm down. In place of fear-adrenalin-sweat, you put acceptance —less adrenalin—less sweat; and finally you have peace—no excess adrenalin—no excess sweat. It is as simple as that, although acceptance may not seem so simple at first.

THE VICAR'S WIFE

Trembling hands are especially difficult to accept when they distribute cups of tea rattling in their saucers to critical guests, as many a vicar's nervous wife has found. I advise any nervous hostess, or secretary, to have the courage to draw attention to her "shakes" and joke about them. If she does, she will find her guests', or her boss's, criticism will change to admiration of her courage, and the "shakes" will soon be taken for granted. Their acceptance encourages her acceptance, and cure will then be well on its way. I have seen this work again and again.

HYPERTHYROIDISM

Hot, trembling hands are also found in a sickness called hyperthyroidism, which is not "just nerves," although it looks very much like it, and which must be specially treated medically. Do not persevere with hot, trembling hands unless you have the assurance of your doctor that you do not have hyperthyroidism. Once given such assurance, accept it and do not waste time and energy worrying for fear the doctor may have made a mistake. If you cannot accept his assurance, seek a second opinion, but do not inquire beyond that. Hyperthyroidism is usually not difficult to diagnose.

RACING HEART OR HEART "SHAKES"

Now examine your racing heart. By "racing" I do not mean the short attacks of palpitation you may have from time to time, but the constantly quickly beating, thumping, banging, "shaking" heart that is your daily companion. You probably think it is racing—that is why I chose this expression—but if you find a watch with a second hand and take your pulse, I doubt if it will be beating at more than a hundred beats each minute. It may be beating at one hundred and twenty, but I doubt even this. In fact, your heart is probably not working much harder than any other healthy heart. The difference is that you have become *sensitized to its beating so that you feel each beat*. And you remain sensitized to its beating while you listen to and anxiously record each beat!

I want you to realize that it will not harm your heart in the least to beat this way. You could play tennis or baseball if you wished. If you had the interest and energy to play such games, it is most likely that your heart would calm down and beat more slowly while you were playing than it does when you are sitting holding your pulse. I am assuming, of course, that you have had a medical examination and have been told that your trouble is "only nerves."

These weeks of waiting, watching, and holding your pulse have been a waste of time. You cannot harm your heart. You can do anything you wish, provided you are prepared to put up temporarily with the strange feelings that come from the region of your heart. The soreness and pain are merely muscular chest-wall strain brought on by tension. A diseased heart does not register pain where you feel it. *Heart pain proper is not felt in the heart.*

So, as far as your heart is concerned, it is a good heart, beating very much like any other. You are only aware of its beating and making yourself more aware by worrying about it and paying it too much attention. Have the courage to relax and analyze this beating and understand that it, too, like the sweating hands and churning stomach, is once again the result of oversensitization of adrenalin-releasing nerves. The nerves of your heart have become so sensitized by fear that they answer the slightest stimulus. A sudden noise may suffice to make your heart "rattle"; or, more puzzling still, it may suddenly beat quickly for no apparent reason.

No Magic Switch

Be prepared to live with this erratic beating until your nerves become less sensitized. They will do this as you become more philosophical and accept the racing and thumping as part of your recovery program. You have made the mistake of thinking that while your heart continued to beat quickly, you must still be ill. It may be some weeks before you will cease to be conscious of its quick action, but once you accept it, *you will be getting better all the time*. There is no magic switch to calm your heart immediately, although sedatives can be a great help and you need not hesitate to let your doctor prescribe them.

SORE SCALP

The soreness around or on top of your head is caused by contraction of your scalp muscles as a result of continuous tension. You may notice how relief comes if you press your scalp or place a hot-water bag where it is most sore. This should prove to you that the cause is local, where you can reach it, and is not deep-seated. *These are not the symptoms of brain tumor*.

Since contraction of tense muscle causes pain, it naturally becomes worse when you worry and improves as you relax and release tension. Pain-killing tablets help, but only a little. With the relaxation that follows acceptance, tension eases and the pain gradually lessens. However, this scalp pain, this "iron band," is a most stubborn symptom to cure, so do not despair if it lingers awhile. I assure you that it eventually goes. The hardest, tightest band will gradually lessen and disappear with acceptance.

"PUTTING UP WITH"

Make sure that you appreciate the difference between truly accepting and only thinking you are accepting. Make sure you know the difference between truly accepting and just "putting up with." "Putting up with" is what you have been doing for a long time. Goodness knows *how* you have been "putting up with," but it hasn't got you very far, has it? "Putting up with" means tensely going forward, hoping the disturbing feelings will not come. "Putting up with" means withdrawing from panic in panic; adding panic to panic, hoping that panic will go quickly and not come back; it means avoiding people and places that bring on panic so that one's horizon becomes narrower and narrower until it is finally bounded by the front gate; it means always keeping the way open for quick retreat; it means expecting retreat. *It means continued illness.*

True acceptance means letting your stomach churn, letting your hands sweat and tremble, letting your heart thump *without being too disconcerted by them.* It does not matter if at first you cannot do this calmly —who could? It may be impossible to be calm at this stage. And you may find that one minute you can accept, the next you can't. Don't be upset by this—it is normal in the circumstances. All I ask for as acceptance at this stage is that *you are prepared* to try to live and work with your symptoms *while they are present,* without paying them too much respect. *Don't be bluffed by physical feelings!*

THE LIMITED POWER OF ADRENALIN-RELEASING NERVES

After examining these "terrible feelings," I want you to remain seated and concentrate on each in turn and try to make it worse. You will find you cannot. *The power of the adrenalin-releasing nerves is limited.* You may succeed in slightly intensifying its effect with concentration, but only slightly. And yet, all the time, without realizing it, you have been shrinking from facing these symptoms squarely because you were afraid that by so doing you would somehow make them worse. It was as if you gave them a fearful, sideways glance.

Let me reassure you. You cannot increase your symptoms by facing them or even trying to intensify them. In fact, you may find that when you try consciously to make them worse, they improve. The very act of concentrating on them in this way means that, for the time being at least, you look at them with some interest rather than fear, and even this brief respite from tension may have a calming effect. In other words, you are no longer withdrawing from your symptoms. *Symptoms can be intensified only by further fear and its resulting tension, never by facing and accepting.* Are you beginning to suspect that your symptoms may have had you bluffed? They most certainly have.

"I CAN'T STAND IT MUCH LONGER!"

A student whose sensations were very much as I have described could make very little headway at his studies because of banging heart, etc. One day, when he thought he would go crazy unless he could get relief, a friend, an ex-soldier, came to see him. He told his friend about his suffering and said, "I can't stand it much longer. I have done all I can to fight it and I don't know which way to turn next. Surely there's a way out of this hell?"

The friend explained that many soldiers at the "front" had had nerves like this until they realized they were only being bluffed by them. He advised the youth to stop being bluffed by his nerves, to float past all suggestion of self-pity and fear, and go on with his work. The student saw the light and, from being afraid to put one foot in front of the other for fear of damaging his heart, in two weeks was climbing mountains. That was many years ago. He has similar feelings now from time to time when overwrought, but he knows that they will pass if he relaxes, goes toward them, accepts, and floats past them. He has learned how to live with his nerves, how to desensitize himself when necessary.

FLOATING

To float is just as important as to accept, and it works similar magic. I could say let "float" and not "fight" be your slogan, because it amounts to that. Just as a person, floating on smooth water, lets himself be carried this way, that way by the gentle movement of the water, so should the nervously ill let his body "go with" the feelings his nervous reactions bring instead of trying to withdraw from them or force his way through them.

Let me illustrate more clearly the practical application of "float." A patient had become so afraid of meeting people that she had not entered a shop for months. When asked to make a small purchase she said, "I couldn't go into a shop. I've tried but I can't. The harder I try, the worse I get. If I force myself, I feel I'm paralyzed and can't put one foot in front of the other. So please don't ask me to go into a shop."

IN DEEP, COOL WATER

I told her that she had little hope of succeeding while she tried to force herself in this way. This was the fighting of which I had previously warned her. Then I showed her a trick I show many patients. I placed my hand on her chest and asked her to move forward against my pressure. When she strained to do this, I pointed out that this was exactly how she had been trying to "conquer" her illness. I then asked her to stretch her arms before her, level with her shoulders, and to move them as if swimming breast stroke. I also asked her to imagine at the same time that she was swimming forward in deep, cool water. I could feel her relax immediately. She also felt the relaxation.

Cannot Take a Bath

I explained that when she stood at the shop door, I wanted her to imagine herself going forward just like that, as if she were gently swimming in, in deep, cool water. This explanation is not popular with nervously ill people who have an aversion to water, even to washing their hair or taking a bath. If you are like this at the moment, don't upset yourself by trying to cope with the thought of "deep, cool water." Choose some other way to "float" that may appeal to you. For instance, the woman I have just been talking about later admitted that she did not like the thought of water, so she imagined she was on a cloud floating through the door.

Bluffed by Thought

I also explained to this woman that she could further help herself by practicing releasing any obstructive thought that might hinder her; practicing letting the thought also "float" away, recognizing that *it was only a thought and she need not be bluffed by a thought,* need not be impressed by a thought.

When she returned she was overjoyed and said, "Don't stop me. I'm still floating. Do you want me to float for something else?"

Strange, isn't it, how the use of one simple word could free a mind that had been imprisoned for months? The explanation is simple enough. When you fight you become tense, and tension inhibits action. When you think of *floating you relax and this helps action.* This woman was in such a state of tension that I have seen her nearly reduced to tears when, with shaking hands, she tried to find a car key in her handbag. After learning to float, one day when on a similar search she said, "Sorry if I'm taking your time. The keys can't be too far away. I've floated past two bills, a lipstick, and a purse. I'll float around a bit longer and find them." The shaking hands were almost steady. She was learning to float past tension.

"Look out, You Might Fall!"

I have seen patients so tensed by continuous fear that they were convinced they could neither walk nor lift their arms to feed themselves. One man afflicted in this way had been bedridden for weeks. After a few conversations with him, I found he was able to understand that the paralysis lay in his thoughts and not in his muscles. He learned the trick of freeing his muscles by *floating past obstructive thought*. Within a few days he was "floating" the food to his mouth unaided, and announced that he was now ready to walk.

This caused a fine stir in the ward. Several doctors, students, and nurses stood by to watch. No sooner had the patient stood up than a nurse, seeing him sway, said hurriedly, "Look out—you might fall!"

The patient, describing the event afterward, said that this suggestion was almost too much and he nearly crumpled to the floor. However, he heard a voice in the background saying, "Float and you can do it. Float past fear," and, he said, "I 'floated' down the hospital ward and back, to my own and everyone else's astonishment."

Such frightening thoughts as were experienced by these two people can be very persistent, almost obsessive, to a tired mind, and it helps some people to imagine a pathway along which they can let these thoughts escape, float away. (Another use for "float.") For example, one woman thought of them as passing out of the back of her head; another said she let them float away along a channel over her right ear, where the grocer keeps his pencil. This may sound childish to a healthy, resilient mind, capable of directing and discarding thought, but to the exhausted, frightened person it is not childish. Nothing that helps is childish to him, and this idea works well.

Masterly Inactivity

Masterly inactivity, a well-known phrase, is another way to describe floating. It means to give up the struggle to stop holding tensely onto yourself, trying to control your fear, trying "to do something about it" while subjecting yourself to constant self-analysis. It means to cease trying to navigate your way out of illness by meeting each obstacle as if it were a challenge that must be met before recovery is possible. It means to bypass the struggle, to go around—not over—the mountain, to float and let time pass.

The average person, tense with battling, has an innate aversion to practicing masterly inactivity and letting go. He vaguely thinks that were he to do this, he would lose control over the last vestige of his will power and his house of cards would tumble. As one young man said, "I feel I must stand on guard. If I were to let go, I'm sure something would snap. It is absolutely necessary for me to keep control and hold myself together." When he was obliged to talk to strangers, he would dig his nails into his palms while he tried to control his trembling body and conceal his state of nervous tension. He would watch the clock anxiously, wondering how much longer he could keep up this masquerade without "cracking."

Loosen Your Attitude

It is especially to such tense, controlled, nail-digging people that I say, "Practice masterly inactivity and let go." If your body trembles, *let it tremble*. Don't feel obliged to try to stop it. Don't try to appear normal. Don't even strive for relaxation. Simply let the thought of relaxation be in your mind, in your attitude toward your body. *Loosen your attitude*. In other words, *don't be too concerned because you are tense and cannot relax*. The very act of being prepared to accept your tenseness relaxes your mind, and relaxation of body gradually follows. You don't have to strive for relaxation. You have to wait for it. When a patient says, "I have tried so hard all day to be relaxed," surely he has had a day of striving, not of relaxation. *Let your body find its own level without controlling it, directing it*. Believe me, if you do this you will not crack. You will not lose control of yourself. You will float up from the depths of despair.

The relief of loosening your tense hold on yourself, of giving up the struggle and recognizing that there is no battle to fight—except of your own making—may bring a calmness you have forgotten existed within you. In your tense effort to control yourself you have been releasing more and more adrenalin and so further exciting your organs to produce the very sensations from which you have been trying to escape.

THE PEAK OF EXPERIENCE

When explaining utter acceptance to a nervously ill person, I stress that this means acceptance *at the very peak of experience.* The following is taken from a taped recording of a conversation with a patient who had been ill for many years.

PATIENT: You knew what was wrong with me. You knew I should try not to tense up when I felt a spell coming; that I should accept and float. And here's the big point. You thought I knew and understood this, but believe me until now I did not. Sure, I accepted most of this and sometimes I was not tense. But at no time, up till now, had I really been fully prepared to accept the way I felt at the climax of my worst suffering.

DOCTOR: At that very moment. *At the peak of experience!* That's the important thing. You thought you were going through with acceptance. You let it come, but at the vital moment you drew back.

PATIENT: Yes. And my apprehension through the day was always of this particular time, dreading it.

DOCTOR: You tried to put up with it. You didn't really accept it.

PATIENT: Sometimes I didn't even put up with it. I withdrew in panic.

DOCTOR: Some people do put up with it better than that, and they think they are accepting, and up to a point they are. They accept 99 per cent, not 100 per cent. It's that extra 1 per cent that makes all the difference. With 100 per cent acceptance, you are prepared to accept *totally* whatever your body, your thoughts may bring, even at the moment of great suffering, above all at this moment. I call this moment *the peak of experience,* and it usually comes at the crest of a wave of panic.

PATIENT: I wasn't doing that. I didn't go along with the effects the tension produced. I ran away. When I mentioned being on guard some weeks ago, I know now that I was on guard to stop myself "listening in" and bringing on a spell. I should have been on guard, ready to relax and accept any spell that might come. It's not that way now. I've learned how to see the spell through without reaching for the pill bottle. I can walk and work even with the panic there. It really doesn't matter any more. It doesn't throw me the way it did. I don't mean that I don't mind having it. It's still horrible, but it just doesn't throw me any more. I've learned what you mean.

> Float past tension and fear.
> Float past unwelcome suggestions.
> Float, don't fight.
> Go through the peak of experience with utter acceptance.
> Let more time pass.

7

Cure of Recurring Nervous Attacks

Now let us consider the symptoms of nervous illness that may occur in attacks—panic spasms, palpitations, slowly beating heart, "missed" heartbeats, trembling spells, a feeling of inability to take a deep breath, "lump in the throat," giddiness, nausea. Depression and sleeplessness are such an important part of nervous illness caused by problem, conflict, sorrow, guilt, or disgrace that to save repetition I shall leave their discussion until describing this second type of nervous illness.

PANIC SPASMS*

As already mentioned, fear can produce a state of constant tension, or it can take the form of intense recurring spasms of panic that start in our "middle" and seem to spread, like a white-hot flame, all over our body, passing through the chest, up the spine, into the face, down the arms, and even into the groin and to the tips of the toes.

If you suffer from these spasms you will probably find that whereas you had some control over them at the beginning of your illness, you now seem to have lost control and live in constant dread of them. Your nerves have become so sensitized that they discharge

---

*Dr. Weekes has made L.P. and cassette recordings in which she talks to you as if she were sitting beside you. Information and recordings available from Galahad Productions, P.O. Box 4996, Washington, D.C. 20008.

panic instantly at the slightest cause. *Feeling follows thought so swiftly it is as if thought and feeling are one.* Sometimes it is almost as if there is no thought, only feeling. This is why a panic spasm may often seem to come unbidden, "out of the blue." Perhaps you will understand more readily if I compare the adrenalin-releasing nerves to the trigger of a gun. When the trigger is rusty, it is hard to pull. When well oiled and used, it responds readily. The nerve trigger in a sensitized person valiantly trying to fight his way through panic is so well used it fires off (and "fire" is a good word) at any encouragement. This is why the sufferer is bewildered, cannot understand what is happening to him; *he used not to be like this.* Of course not. He has not always been sensitized.

ANALYZING FEAR. TWO SEPARATE FEARS

Cure lies in desensitization, and there is no doubt that the key to desensitization lies in learning *how to cope with panic.* Recurring panic, more than any other nervous symptom, helps to keep nervous illness alive. To cope with panic it is important for the nervously ill person to understand that when he panics, he feels not one fear, as he supposes, but *two separate fears.* Because his nerves are sensitized, one fear follows the other so swiftly *it is as if the two fears are one.* With each wave of panic there are always *two separate fears involved.* I call these the *first* and *second* fears.

The importance of recognizing these two separate fears cannot be overestimated, because although the nervously ill person, as a result of sensitization, may have no direct control over the *first* fear, with understanding and practice he can learn how to control *second* fear, and *it is this second fear that is keeping the first fear alive, keeping him sensitized, keeping him nervously ill.*

First fear

I will explain these two separate fears more fully. Everyone experiences *first* fear from time to time. It is the fear that comes reflexly, almost automatically, in response to some threatened danger. It is normal in intensity—we understand it, we accept it. We cope with the danger and the fear passes. However, the flash of *first* fear that comes to a sensitized person in response to danger is not normal in intensity. It can be so overwhelmingly intense, so electric in its swiftness, so out of proportion to the danger causing it that a sensitized person cannot readily dismiss it. Indeed, he usually immediately recoils from it, and as he does this he adds a second flash of fear to the first flash. He adds fear of the first flash. Indeed, he may be much more concerned with the physical feeling of panic than with the original danger. And because that old bogy, sensitization, prolongs the first flash, the second flash may actually seem to join it. This is why the two fears so often feel as one.

A flash of *first* fear may follow no more than the sudden impact of a cold blast of wind. It may follow merely some mildly unpleasant memory; it may come in response to a thought only vaguely understood, or, as I mentioned earlier, it may seem to come "out of the blue." Can you see how susceptible a sensitized person could so easily become to that *first* flashing fear? And he is particularly susceptible to *first* fear when he is hemmed in by people, such as at a school gathering, in church.

"Oh, my goodness! Here it is again!"

A nervously ill person has only to think of being trapped for *first* fear to flash instantly. To this he immediately adds plenty of *second* fear as he thinks "Oh, my goodness! Here it is again! I can't stand it. I'll make a fool of myself in front of all these people. Let me out of here. Quickly! Quickly!" With each "Quickly!" he adds more and more panic, more and more tension, and as the tension mounts, naturally the panic mounts in intensity, until he is never quite sure just how intense the panic can become or what crisis it may bring. He is sure there must be a crisis in which he vaguely imagines himself being taken off "somewhere."

This hovering threat holds such menace that at the peak of panic the sufferer thinks he can no longer think clearly or act calmly. This is why he sits near the door at the restaurant, at the back of the school meeting, so that he can (as I have already mentioned) slip out unnoticed if his fears seem to grow beyond him. He does not understand that it is the fears he adds himself, the succession of *second* fears, that may finally drive him to find refuge outside the building. He doesn't understand that it is all those Oh, my goodnesses, all those What ifs that build up into what he calls a spell, a crisis. If he could but realize that his body is not a machine, that it has a limited capacity to produce adrenalin, that therefore the *first* fear can come only in a wave and must always die down, *if he but waits* and does not fall into the trap of stoking his fires with *second* fear.

No mounting panic

If he were prepared to sit in his seat, relax his body to the best of his ability—let it sag, flop into his seat —and *let the panic flash,* let it *do its very worst,* let it flash right through him without withdrawing tensely from it, *there would be no mounting tension, no mounting panic.* His sensitized body may continue to flash panic for a while, *but the panic would not mount,* and he would be able to sit there and see the function through.

Also, it is bombardment by *second* fear, day after day, week after week, for one excuse or another that keeps nerves alerted, always triggered to fire that *first* fear so sensitively, flashingly, electrically when under stress.

Unmask that second fear

How important it is to unmask panic and see those two separate fears. How important it is to learn how to spot *second* fear and send it packing. Recognizing *sec-*

ond fear and coping with it is the way to desensitization, the way to recovery. I assure you of this. Recognizing *second* fear is made easier when we realize that it can usually be prefixed by "Oh, my goodness!" and "What if . . . ?" "Oh, my goodness. It took four capsules to get me to sleep last night. What if four don't work tonight?" "Oh, my goodness, what if I get worse, not better?" So many Oh, my goodnesses, so many What ifs make up that *second* fear.

Now, just as you examined and described your churning stomach, sweating hands, etc., on the next occasion when you panic I want you to examine this feeling, describing it to yourself as it sweeps through you.

Only a bogy remains

Must you let a physical feeling hold such terror? Must you let a hot feeling in your stomach, a burning flash up your spine, pins and needles in your hands, a throbbing feeling in your head, even a weak feeling in your legs spoil life? Think about this and realize *you are being bluffed by physical feeling,* terrible indeed, but still a *physical feeling!*

All the symptoms that come with stress, the pounding heart, churning stomach, weak feelings, etc., can be called *first* fears because they, too, come unbidden like the flash of fear that comes in answer to danger; and to these symptoms the nervously ill person certainly adds plenty of *second* fear, certainly adds many Oh, my goodnesses, many What ifs, more than enough to keep his fires well burning. Oh, yes; he adds plenty of *second* fear to these symptoms.

By analyzing fear and its symptoms in this way and seeing them as physical feelings that conform to a set pattern and are of no great medical significance, you unmask fear and with it your own illness, and *only a bogy remains*. And when you decide to accept this bogy and add no more *second* fear (or as little as you can manage) the road to recovery lies open before you. Now, even with great success at learning how to cope with *second* fear, it takes time for desensitization. The nervously ill person must understand and accept that his sensitized body will flash *first* fear from time to time for some time to come. If you are like this, I assure you that if you do not continue to whip your sensitized body with *second* fear, it will heal its sensitized nerves as naturally as it would heal a broken leg. *But this takes time.* To face and accept one's nervous symptoms without adding *second* fear and to let time pass for recovery—how important this is. It works miracles if you are prepared to do just this.

But it is not easy to face, accept, and let time pass. It is especially difficult to let time pass, because you may already have let so much time pass in suffering and despair that asking you to let more time pass may seem an impossible demand. It is difficult but necessary.

Also, don't think I underestimate the severity of your panic. I know how severe it can be and I also know that even with the help of daily sedation and the best of intentions and determination to accept it, you may think yourself too exhausted to do so. It is as if your mind is ready to accept but your body is so tired that you cannot make it accept. As one woman said, "I can't seem to get a 'holt' on it, Doctor."

CONTINUOUS SEDATION

If like this you may need complete rest in the form of continuous sleep for a few days. This is achieved by supervised sedation, which we call "continuous sedation." This sounds gruesome to some patients, who shrink from the thought of it. They see themselves lost to the world for days in a state of coma, like the hypnotized man in the shop window. It is not like that. Your doctor, and nobody else, prescribes a sedative to ensure sleep at night. On waking the next morning you bathe and have breakfast as usual and then take another dose of sedative for further sleep. After lunch, you may sleep without additional sedative. If not, more is given. This regime continues for a few days, or even a few weeks, if necessary.

Let your doctor prescribe

Remember, if you need sedatives even in small doses, you must let your doctor prescribe and supervise the dosage. Do not buy them over the counter at the drugstore. Some proprietary lines have dangerous side effects of which the pharmacist may be unaware.

"Only one pill last night, Doctor!"

You need not fear addiction from supervised sedation. When you are well you will not need sedatives. People with nervous illness seem to take a particular delight in doing without sedatives as soon as possible. They may try to do without them too soon. How many times have I been greeted with a triumphant, "Only one pill last night, Doctor!"

Sedation is particularly necessary if you cannot sleep, because sleep is such an excellent healer. However, sleep is of most value when it is accompanied by peace of mind. If you have accepted the strange feelings and are no longer running away from them, you will have found some peace. Sleep will now be a boon. But sleep is less helpful to the person who stays afraid and keeps mentally running away. However, even here, sleep has some restorative power, and we rely on this when we advise continuous sedation to a particularly distressed, exhausted person.

OTHER WAYS TO CONQUER FEAR

There are ways to conquer fear other than analyzing and unmasking it, and some doctors have the experience of watching a sufferer inventing his own method. Some find the cause of the fear and try to conquer and control it, believing that with the cause removed the fear will go. For example, one woman, terrified of the palpitations because of fear of dying during an attack, so succeeded in losing her fear of death that she lost her fear of the palpitations. I have not suggested that you use this method for this type of illness, because there are too many instances where much would be made from nothing, and one difficulty overcome only to find a dozen in its place. At this stage I prefer to attack fear itself.

THE NEIGHBOR WITH THE GLITTERING EYE

For example, Mrs. G. was afraid to walk up the street to go shopping. When she analyzed why she was afraid, she found many obstacles causing fear, among them passing the telephone booth where she had once collapsed, passing the neighbor with the glittering eye, waiting to be served at the butcher's, and so on—the list was long. To discover why she feared each obstacle would have been a research program in itself. Common sense rebels at the thought. It is more satisfactory to find a common approach to meet each obstacle encountered on that journey up the street. Unmasking fear itself is such an approach. No longer afraid of the physical sensation of fear, Mrs. G. can float past the telephone booth, past the neighbor's glittering eye, even into the butcher's.

While this method is excellent for minor fears, major fears must indeed be attacked at their source, otherwise unmasking fear is only dodging the issue. By major fear I mean a fear big enough to have originally caused illness and to be now interfering with recovery. I have reserved consideration of such a sufferer for another chapter.

PALPITATIONS

This short attack of alarmingly quickly beating heart may come, and so often does, just as you are going off to sleep, or may even wake you from sleep. Do not sit up in panic. The more you panic, the more adrenalin is released by your glands and nerves and the quicker your heart beats. Although you may think, "Ah, I wish the doctor could feel my pulse now! My heart really is racing!" I still suspect that if you take your own pulse you will find that its rate is not much more than one hundred and twenty beats to each minute.

Even if it is, it is not important. A healthy heart can tolerate a rate of over two hundred beats per minute for many hours, even days, without evidence of damage.

How Thick and Powerful Is Your Heart Muscle

Also, you may think you can feel your heart beating in your throat and are sure it will burst at any moment. I can assure you it will not. The full, bursting feeling is no more than the unusually hard pumping of the main arteries in your neck. Your heart is nowhere near your throat. If you could see how thick and appreciate how powerful your heart muscle is, you would lose all fear of its bursting or being damaged by the palpitations. I must remind you that I am assuming that your doctor has examined your heart and has told you that your trouble is "nerves."

So relax to the best of your ability (see "How to Relax" in Chapter 20) and let your heart race until it chooses to slow down, remembering that it is a good heart, merely temporarily overstimulated, and that such stimulation will not harm it and will soon cease. Should the attack be prolonged, does it matter so much? When you understand the palpitations, are they so terrible? If necessary you can ease yourself by talking to someone or getting up and drinking a glass of milk. Walking about will not harm your heart even though it is palpitating. If you prefer to stay in bed, by all means do so, but lie there as relaxed as possible and let your heart race *without shrinking from it*. If you do this, one of these nights you will surprise yourself by dropping off to sleep in the middle of an attack.

As acceptance calms your nerves, the attacks will be less frequent until they no longer come. Many years ago when studying under strain, I occasionally had palpitations. I have not had an attack since. Can you see how foolish it would have been had I become agitated by them? My heart has served me well during the ensuing thirty years.

SLOWLY BEATING HEART

It may be that instead of beating too quickly, your heart occasionally beats too slowly for comfort and you have attacks of faintness, when you are sure it is about to stop altogether. In such an attack you may feel paralyzed, unable to move. This is called a vasovagal attack and is brought on by overstimulation of the parasympathetic nerve, the vagus. You will remember that the parasympathetic nerves hold the adrenalin-releasing nerves in check. In these attacks they check too severely and the heart slows to an uncomfortable rate.

Vasovagal attacks are rarer than palpitations, but they are just as disturbing if you do not understand them. Remember, the attack is also the result of *too much nervous stimulation. Your heart is not diseased. The attack does not harm your heart.* As you worry less, sustained tension lessens and the attacks gradually leave you. Even after apparent recovery, you may occasionally have one. Do not be disconcerted by this. With understanding and acceptance they seem less formidable. Actually, your doctor can prescribe tablets to control them, so consult him if necessary. It is well to terminate an attack quickly, as it can be exhausting although not actually harmful. Although I teach facing and accepting, I do not advocate stoical forbearance.

"MISSED" HEARTBEATS

A nervously tired heart, a heart stimulated by too much alcohol, nicotine, caffeine (coffee, tea), irritated by indigestion, will sometimes "miss" beats. The sufferer describes it as "missing" beats, although no beat is actually missed. The heartbeats are merely spaced unevenly. The patient feels as if his heart turns over and a tickling sensation catches him in the throat. He may cough and stand still, wondering what will happen next.

"Missed" beats are in no way dangerous, and your

heart will not stop because of them. They are annoying but that is all. *Exercise abolishes them.* So do not let "missed" beats frighten you into lying on the couch again. Most people over forty have "missed" beats now and then. Many young people have them. *They are not important.*

TREMBLING TURNS

Some people have weak turns that are neither palpitations nor attacks of slowly beating heart. They refer to them as "trembling turns" and describe how their legs suddenly feel weak and tremble and their body breaks out into a clammy sweat. They do not actually faint, although they may feel they will. The attack gradually passes on resting. These are called hypoglycemic attacks, and that long word means merely "not enough sugar in the blood." In other words, the engine is knocking for lack of gasoline.

Hypoglycemic attacks come especially to tense people who use their supply of energy faster than they can replenish. The attack usually occurs before meals and is quite harmless. Resting alone will end it, as the liver then releases sugar into the blood stream. Eating something sweet helps the attack to pass quickly. It is a good idea to keep some sweets handy. These attacks are not restricted to people with nervous illness. Many energetic, healthy people have them.

INABILITY TO TAKE A DEEP BREATH

Just as tension causes scalp muscles to spasm and pain, so does it cause chest and lung muscles to spasm and the patient to complain that he cannot expand his chest sufficiently to take in a deep breath. He may walk around the house sighing until asked by an exasperated relative to "Please stop those lamentations."

The effect of such spasm is temporary and is released with relief from tension. It does not harm your chest. Your chest is not diseased. You will always get enough breath, although sometimes perhaps not as freely as you would like.

Let Your "Breathing Center" Do the Work

Some patients are so afraid they will suffocate that they struggle and fight for breath, believing that unless they win the battle the end is near. I explain to these people that nature was not so careless as to put such a responsibility in their hands. How do they think they breathe while asleep? This question never fails to surprise them.

We have a "breathing center" in our brain which automatically regulates our breathing by responding to changing levels of carbon dioxide in our blood. To illustrate how this center works, I ask one of these apprehensive people to see how long he can hold his breath, how long he can actually stop breathing. To his surprise he finds that after about half a minute he is forced to breathe again. When he realizes that there is a control beyond his control waiting to protect him, he begins to see the folly of struggling so desperately to "take a deep breath." He should breathe as shallowly as he feels he must and not be so concerned with what will happen. He can safely rely on his respiratory center to cope with the difficulty in its own way. It will not fail him.

Blow into a Paper Bag

Shallow breathing may have one harmless, yet frightening effect. The nervously ill person may breathe so rapidly in his misguided effort to get enough air into his lungs that he may temporarily wash out too much carbon dioxide from his lungs. He may then feel giddy, and his hands, charged with "pins and needles," may stiffen and flex at the wrist. This is alarming to patient and family but is so harmless that simply breathing into a paper bag and then rebreathing the expired air for a few minutes ends the attack.

"LUMP IN THE THROAT"

Some nervous people complain that they feel a constant pressure in the throat or that they have a "lump

stuck in the throat," which they keep trying to dis-
lodge by swallowing. Some say that their throats seem
"swollen inside." These patients are convinced that
there is something seriously wrong with them, even
cancer. Once again we are merely concerned with muscular spasm of nervous origin. We call this globus
hystericus, which means the hysterical lump. It, too,
will vanish with relaxation and acceptance, although
in the meantime it can be so aggravating that the
person afflicted finds it difficult to believe that such a
definite feeling of pressure can be only spasm. It is not
always easy to convince him of the nervous origin of
his "lump," and he is reassured only after the doctor
has made a thorough examination of his throat.

GIDDINESS

Giddiness can be a most upsetting phenomenon. To
us, the stability of our world depends very much on
seeing it as we are accustomed. Suddenly to have the
impression that the furniture is speeding across the
room can indeed be an alarming experience.

Giddiness is of two main types. In one, objects we
know to be stationary may seem to move; in the other,
we may simply feel unsteady, lightheaded. Our balance is normally maintained by such complex muscular
co-ordination between eyes, ears, and eye and neck
muscles that the slightest deviation from normal may
make us sway and feel giddy. So you will appreciate
that giddiness may be an early visitor to a fatigued
nervous system, although an unimportant one, since it
comes only in brief attacks and vanishes quickly with
regained composure and loss of fatigue.

As certain small physical defects can cause giddiness,
such as a piece of wax stuck to an eardrum or a
blocked Eustachian tube (the tube that passes from the
ear to the throat), it is as well to have your doctor's assurance that your giddiness is due to "nerves." Nervous
giddiness is usually the lightheaded type. The nervously
ill person finds himself unsteady, off balance.

NAUSEA

Eating may be a problem. You have probably lost weight and feel nauseated at the sight of food. Do not make the mistake of thinking that because you feel nauseated and are under stress, your food is doing you little good and that therefore you need not eat much. Even when eaten in these conditions food will nourish you, although it may take longer than normal to digest. Malnutrition and anemia can bring symptoms like yours, *so you must eat enough*.

If you have eaten poorly for weeks, your stomach may be unable at first to hold a normal-sized meal. If so, take small meals frequently. Drink egg flips and plenty of milk. Also, take a daily dose of vitamins, but only the amount prescribed by a doctor. Too many vitamins can be as dangerous as too few.

DIFFICULTY IN SWALLOWING

The "lump in the throat" described earlier may be most troublesome at mealtime. The sufferer is sure he cannot swallow solid food, or at least finds this difficult.

"I'll Never Get It Down!"

I keep biscuits in my office especially for such a patient. Biscuits are dry, and at the sight of one the patient usually recoils. When I ask him to chew one, he says, "I couldn't swallow a biscuit. I'd never get it down!" I remind him that I asked him to chew, not swallow. Reluctantly he bites and chews. After a while I say, "Now remember, I want you only to chew. Don't swallow." But already he has swallowed some of it. As soon as the moistened, softened biscuit reaches the back of his tongue, his swallowing reflexes take over and at least some of the biscuit is on its way.

You need not worry about trying to *swallow;* simply keep *chewing.* The swallowing will look after itself as the food is carried backward. And it will eventually find its way backward in spite of your nervous resistance. If you keep chewing, the food will all eventually disappear.

FEAR OF VOMITING

Many nervously ill people are haunted by fear of vomiting in public, but I have not yet met one who has actually done this. Many have gagged gently to themselves or have hurriedly left the hall to gag in the lane outside, but vomit food—no. This is remarkable when we realize that short of putting his finger down his throat, a nervous person could hardly stimulate his stomach, abdominal, and throat muscles more than he does by his tense, anxious control of them. It is not as easy for a healthy stomach to vomit food as one imagines.

If the nervously ill person were to let go and give up the struggle to try not to vomit, his muscles would gradually relax and vomiting would be even less likely. If he does not vomit while tensely on guard, he certainly will not do so when he relaxes and lowers that guard, and how much more comfortable he will be.

LOSING WEIGHT: KEEP OFF THOSE SCALES

Provided you are practicing accepting and letting time pass and are eating your meals, especially that last extra bit you don't want, *your weight is not important*. People with nervous illness place unnecessary significance on losing weight. They view their protruding bones with growing alarm, wondering just how far the fading-away process can go before they fall to pieces completely. They haunt the bathroom scales, eyes glued to the dial, while they try to jiggle out a few extra ounces. *Cover your scales and resist all temptation to stand on them until you are so fat that you think it is time to diet.*

It is interesting to note the direct and yet temporary effect of emotional stress on appetite. I have seen a distressed person gag at the sight of food, only to devour it ravenously an hour later after hearing good news.

The body made thin by fear is not diseased and is

waiting to recover lost weight as soon as you will pass
the food down to it. So place no importance on your
wasted looks, your "poor thin body." *Eat up and forget
those scales.* Even when some cheerful friend says,
"Good heavens, you are thinner than ever!" still resist
the temptation to step onto the scales.

No Permanent Damage

Indeed, when your neighbor gives you a pitying
glance and says, "You look awful!" remember that
however ill you may appear today, in a few weeks the
same neighbor could be saying, "You *do* look different!" *You can recover completely from your nervous
illness.* You will not be left with a damaged heart, in
spite of the pains you may now feel in that region.

So why not think, "I may look awful today, but nervous illness is not a disease. As soon as I am a little
better, I will put on more weight. In the meantime I'll
eat up, even if I have to push the food down, or chew
it for hours, and I'll float past my neighbor's com-
ments."

NO NEW SYMPTOMS CAN ARISE

It may comfort you to know that *the action of
adrenalin is always restricted to the same organs and
so must always follow the same pattern. There are no
more surprises in store for you.* This thought comforts
most people because apprehension of what can happen
next is a big part of their illness. *Other than the symptoms already described, no new symptoms of any significance can arise.*

If you have had only some of the symptoms mentioned, do not immediately think you must now experience all the others. It is unusual to have all the symptoms. Each of us has some parts of his body more
sensitive than the rest, and which therefore react more
readily to stimulation by adrenalin. If you have not
been nauseated, it is because your stomach is strong
enough to withstand tension. It should continue to do
so. We all know that certain people have a tendency to

"heave" when upset, others to run to the toilet, while others just churn inwardly. Few do all three.

Your particular pattern has probably declared itself by now, so you can be comforted by the thought that you have experienced the worst.

8

Fear of Leaving the Safety of Home (Agoraphobia)

Most people have heard of claustrophobia (fear of enclosed places), but very few have heard of agoraphobia, a much more crippling illness. Agoraphobia, a Greek word meaning "fear of the market place," in actual practice means fear of leaving the safety of home, either alone or in the company of others. This includes fear of traveling far from home, of entering shops, and sometimes even fear of walking to the end of the street to mail a letter.

Most people with claustrophobia speak frankly of their fear, but people with agoraphobia rarely admit to their condition. They will find excuse after excuse to avoid visiting friends, going here, going there. I have known women suffering with agoraphobia whose own husbands do not know about it, so well have they camouflaged their fears. Very few who suffer this way know that their illness has a name and that thousands of other people suffer as they do. It has been estimated that in England alone one hundred thousand people suffer with agoraphobia today. In America, with its far greater population, there must be many more than this.

Agoraphobia is comparatively common because it develops so naturally from an anxiety state. A frightened, sensitized person tries to stay where she feels safe, or where she thinks she can get help quickly if she needs it.

She Avoids and Avoids and Avoids

I speak now of woman rather than man, because more women than men suffer from fear of leaving the safety of home. A woman's life at home is more conducive to the development of this phase of nervous illness. She avoids putting herself in situations where she feels she may have a spell. So she begins to avoid and avoid and avoid, until to put one foot before the other in the street, if alone, may be a misery. Agoraphobia is simple enough to understand when we see it like this. There is no mystery here, and how human it all is.

Since this woman is afraid of having a spell when she is out, she is more likely to have one when she is out, because a spell is no more than she, herself, frightening herself. How could she not panic when she is so afraid of panicking? She prepares the way for panic before she leaves the house. This is why going out is such a strain. As I have explained so often, panic may flash so suddenly in a sensitized person that it may seem to come out of the blue. This is what bewilders, amazes, frightens. And this is why her horizon may finally be bounded by her front door.

I will not use the term "agoraphobia" again. It labels fear too definitely and makes it sound too discouragingly permanent.

"It All Started after the Birth of My Baby"

If you are suffering from fear of leaving the safety of home, you possibly had an experience in the past that upset you to an exaggerated extent and, as I have already explained, sensitized you. So many mothers say, "It all started after the birth of my last baby."

If like this, you are not really afraid of wide open spaces, or of the "market place" ("supermarket," today). You know perfectly well that if you go to the corner store, the grocer won't shoot you, the houses won't fall upon you. You know none of these things will harm you. So what are you afraid of? You are afraid of the feelings that arise within you when you are in this situation, feelings that seem to overwhelm you so that you seem unable to think clearly while they are present. You don't trust yourself while you are like this, and this is why you are afraid to go out by yourself.

I Will Take You by the Hand

I am now going to take you out with me, step by step, and as we go I will explain exactly what happens, why it happens, and what to do about it. Are you ready? Good.

Your First Mistake

But look at you. Before we've opened the front door, you have tensed yourself like a violin string screwed up tightly. You thought, "Oh, my goodness! What's going to happen now?" If one plucks a taut violin string, it responds by vibrating, whereas a slack string does not. By tensing your body, you made of it an instrument on which your fears can play a very painful tune, and you did this before you even put one foot outside your door. *This is your first mistake.*

Instead of tensing your body in anticipation of what may happen, let it go, slacken it, release it. *Slacken those strings.* The worst that can happen to you out there in the street, in the shop, is that you can let yourself become frightened. *I know how severe that fright can be,* but if you release as much tension as possible and are prepared to accept what happens, prepared to surrender yourself to it, it won't be quite so overwhelming. Surrender, accept. Slacken those strings. Take a slow breath, let it out gently. Have you the idea? Good.

Here Comes Mrs. X

We are off. But, oh, my goodness, here comes Mrs. X from down the street. What are you going to do about her? You advance toward her with "your heart in your mouth." You can feel your heart thumping in your throat, banging in your chest. But your neighbor's heart is also beating quickly, perhaps just as quickly as yours. She's excited because she hasn't seen you for weeks out alone. Then why should your heart's quick beating be so especially frightening? So particularly uncomfortable? Your sensitized nerves are recording and amplifying every beat. Does it matter if you feel your heart beating? It doesn't matter in the least. It certainly doesn't harm your heart. So don't be afraid to feel your heart beat while you talk to Mrs. X.

A GOOD OLD GOSSIP

But she is settling in for a good old gossip. What if she were to continue for another ten minutes, *half an hour?* You tremble at the thought and think "I can't stand it. I'll make a fool of myself. She'll notice!"

But now I whisper, "Take your hand off that screw. Let your body go slack. Loosen. Loosen. Take a slow breath, let it out slowly and surrender completely to listening to Mrs. X. She'll eventually stop."

You hear me. You hesitate and then you release the tension just a little, and, strangely enough, when you do that, standing there does not seem quite so difficult. You even feel a little pleased with yourself. And so you should, because you have discovered something very important. You've learned that Mrs. X. is not upsetting you, as you thought; *you were upsetting yourself. It was your hand tightening that screw, not hers.*

CROSSING THE MAIN ROAD

Now we're off down the street again. You feel a little better. You made it! But now you must cross the main road, and just when you need your legs most they suddenly turn to jelly. Those old, jelly legs. Did I say suddenly? It didn't happen quite so suddenly as you thought. As you approached the main road, you became frightened again, and fear released that old enemy adrenalin, which gave you the jelly legs. When we inject adrenalin into a person suffering with asthma, his legs feel weak and he may sit down until the reaction passes. This is a normal process. Your legs are responding normally to the adrenalin you gave yourself when you were afraid. The effect will gradually pass if you do not become frightened of it and so add more adrenalin. But you don't know this and you stand rooted to the pavement, sure that your legs will never carry you across.

JELLY LEGS WILL STILL GET YOU THERE

But here again I whisper, "Jelly legs will still get you there if you will let them. It is only a feeling. Not a true weakness. Don't be bluffed by jelly legs. And don't add more adrenalin by being afraid of them. Let them wobble. They'll get you across the street whether they wobble or not. And don't think you have to hold tensely on to yourself to keep yourself from collapsing. It's the holding on that exhausts, not the letting go. So let your legs wobble. It's only a feeling, not a true muscular weakness."

You crossed the road. You made it. By now you are not quite so impressed by the tricks your body has been playing on you. When you realize this you somehow feel charged with new strength. But wait! You had forgotten about the store! There may be half a dozen neighbors ready to talk in there. You may even have to wait in a line.

THE FULL FEAR TREATMENT

In a flash you turn on all screws at once and give yourself the full fear treatment. It is as if you have made no progress at all, and just when you thought you were beginning to get the right idea. And while you look at the shop in despair your body seems to sway, the street to swirl, the buildings to topple, everything goes blurred. You clutch at a post to steady yourself. How are we going to explain this one? *This* is a beauty.

It is explained very simply. Severe tension disturbs co-ordination between your muscles and your balancing apparatus, and this apparatus receives the wrong messages, so the buildings seem to topple and you feel unsteady. Also fear dilates your pupils and vision therefore seems blurred. This is so frightening that you withdraw from it and let it overwhelm you. But it is only the same old tricks in disguise, the same old turn of the screw. And as usual you turned it yourself.

LET THE STORM PASS

Wait! Let the storm pass. Let the effects of adrenalin pass. Even at the climax to your fears, surrender and accept. At the very moment when your feelings seem to engulf you, that is the moment above all when you must surrender and accept. No more Oh, my goodnesses, no more What ifs. If you do this, you will find that you will keep that grip on yourself you previously always seemed to lose. If you go forward, *however hesitatingly,* with understanding of what is happening, ready to accept all the tricks your fears may play upon you, your reactions will gradually calm and you won't have to wear dark glasses, or push a baby carriage for support, when you go out (some of you suffer enough to resort to these subterfuges); you won't have to try walking as far as the corner store one day, into town the next, until you finally graduate to the supermarket. You will find peace in the middle of Times Square, *because you will take your cure with you wherever you might be.*

TAKE YOURSELF BY THE HAND

Just as you read this advice now, say it to yourself again and again when you are out until you make it part of yourself. It will never fail you if you follow it and follow it until you learn to take yourself by the hand, until you are your own guide, your own strength.

LONG-PLAYING RECORDS

To help people who are recovering by using this book, I have made an album of two long-playing records on special aspects of nervous illness. In these records I talk especially about panic and how to deal with it, including fear of leaving the safety of home and fear of being alone. There is also a long section on Coming through Setback. (See footnote on page 196.)

9

Being Yourself Again

Having faced and accepted the disturbing sensations of nervous illness, your next question will be, "How long before I am myself again?" Now, it is almost certain that, despite your new approach to your illness, your symptoms will continue to return for some time —perhaps, at first, as acutely as before you read this book. You will understand this when you appreciate that your adrenalin-releasing nerves will continue to be fatigued and sensitized for some time longer, in spite of the new approach.

I often find that after talking for the first time to a nervously ill patient, he leaves the consulting room elated and convinced he is cured, sure that he has found the magic wand at last, only to return a few days later, disappointed and depressed, in spite of a warning that this could happen. I explain again that his nerves need more time to respond to the new approach; that he is like a runner in a race who, having touched the goal and won the race, must continue to run some yards before he can stop. When these people finally understand and accept this, they take heart. Understanding and willingness to let more time pass finally work the miracle.

Calm acceptance, *despite delayed recovery,* is your goal. However, although you understand and try to accept calmly, at first you may find calm acceptance very difficult. Do not be disappointed. In the beginning it is enough to direct your thoughts toward acceptance. Calm acceptance will follow in time.

Also, it may be that although you wish to be unafraid, you may still add plenty of *second* fear. Do not be discouraged even by this. *If you can but understand what I have been teaching you,* you have made the first step toward recovery. It is enough at this stage *to wish to be unafraid.* Provided you make up your mind *to accept the strange feelings although still afraid of them,* you will gradually lose your fear, because decision to accept releases a certain tension and so reduces the intensity of your symptoms. This brings a little hope, and you begin to gain confidence in recovery. Loss of fear eventually follows.

THE FRONT LINE OF BATTLE

Do not think I expect you to do this without the help of sedation. When you go out ready to face and accept, you willingly put yourself in the front line of battle, as it were, for the time being, and you may feel plenty of panic, feel nervier than ever, be temporarily more sensitized. You may therefore need extra tranquilization while you go through the early stages of recovery. It is necessary to find the dose that helps to tranquilize without making you lethargic or depressed. You must have a doctor's help in choosing the type and dose of sedative. However, do not persist in taking the dose if it seems too heavy. Use your common sense. It is sometimes difficult to select accurately the amount to suit a particular person. Trial does this. So do not hesitate to lessen your dose if you so desire. However, do not increase it without your doctor's consent.

KEEP OCCUPIED

It is essential that you be occupied while awaiting cure. However, I must warn you against *feverishly seeking occupation in order to forget yourself*. This is running away from fear, and you can't run far from fear. I want you to be occupied while facing your symptoms and to accept the possibility of their return from time to time during recovery. There is a world of difference between these two approaches. It is as if you halt your feverish rushing, relax and walk more calmly, thinking to yourself, "All right! Let the feelings come. Running away won't prevent them. But if I accept them, they will gradually calm down. In the meantime, I'll keep my mind occupied with work, so that I need not think of them unnecessarily."

Every short respite from fear helps to calm your nerves so that they become less and less responsive to stimulation and your sensations less and less intense, until they are only a memory.

QUICK RECOVERY

I once wrote to a friend in a sanatorium, advising her how to recover from her nervous illness. Some months later, a stranger telephoned to thank me for the letter, which my friend had shown her. This woman said she knew she was cured before she finished reading it, and had been able to leave the hospital within a few days. She said that now, four months later, she was still cured and was confident she would never relapse. Complete understanding was her shield.

Such quick recovery is possible, and when I say you may continue to feel fear and the persistence of symptoms for some time and must be prepared to let more time pass, do not misunderstand and think that I mean that all recovery from illness is a long-drawn-out process. Recovery can be, as just illustrated, dramatically quick. I have merely warned you that your recovery may not be as rapid as you expect, so that you will not be unnecessarily disappointed. "Letting more time pass" means no more than being patient a little longer, but I purposely have not asked directly for patience, because the thought of being patient may seem an impossibility to a sufferer from highly tensed nerves. For this reason I chose the phrase, "let more time pass." The difference is subtle but important. Where the sufferer is prepared to let more time pass, he may think he could not take advice to be patient. The very sound of the word is exasperating.

GRADUAL RECOVERY

Physical exhaustion may delay recovery, but, even here, with good food and peace of mind, two or three months are usually long enough to reclaim a person from a nervous illness of some severity, provided he does not have too many setbacks. Each patient recovers at his own pace, and this depends on the rate of returning confidence and peace of mind. *The strength in a limb may depend on the confidence with which it is used.* When you appreciate that wrong thinking can "paralyze" some people and keep them bedridden, you will understand how hesitant, diffident thinking can encourage weakness. Returning confidence and physical strength go hand in hand.

Mrs. L. had been attending a gymnasium weekly for three years where instructors, interested in the treatment of functional nervous disorders, were so anxious that their clients should not overtax their physical strength, and so insistent that recovery must be gradual, that this woman, after three years, had little confidence in her own strength and was prepared to wait even longer for it to return fully.

After I had pointed out that her real trouble was lack of confidence and not muscular weakness and explained that she must free herself from thought paralysis and use her muscles to strengthen them, she surprised herself by the amount she could do in a few days. She said, "I'm amazed. I only thought I couldn't do these things. It doesn't seem possible that wrong thinking could have kept me so weak, but it has!" I had a card from her recently and she said, "I'm still using the golden key you gave me, and nobody can see my heels for dust!"

Do not watch the calendar and time your recovery. Let time pass, as little or as much as necessary.

Let the pace of your recovery look after itself.

Be concerned only with recognizing and coping with *second* fear and the use of your muscles.

THE OLD FORGOTTEN SENSATIONS

When I review the difficulties of recovery, I would say that the most alarming of them all is the way panic can flash so intensely, so quickly and unexpectedly— weeks, months, even years—after a person thinks he has completely recovered. This unexpected return of panic causes more concern than any other aspect of nervous illness; it shocks, it frightens, and *it reminds*—that is why it is so shocking. It reminds of so much one would rather forget forever, of so much one thought one had forgotten. And the fear that is immediately added, to- gether with the physical disturbance caused by the flash of panic, resensitizes slightly and brings back some of the old, almost forgotten sensations of nervous illness, so that the unwary sufferer is often bluffed into thinking "it" has returned, or that "it" will return if he doesn't watch out.

BACK TO THE SAFETY OF HOME

Almost invariably he makes the old mistake of ca- pitulating before the feeling and trying to run away from it, watching "over his shoulder" for fear it comes again. One woman who had a return of panic while shopping immediately dashed back home and then avoided that particular shop for weeks. She made the mistake of retreating from fear in fear once more.

Never do this. Never let the unexpected return of panic, whenever it may strike—even if it comes years after you think it has gone forever—never let it shock you into running away from it. *Halt.* Go slowly. See the panic through and then quietly go on with what you are doing. Let the panic come again and again if it should.

SOME STRAIN, SOME TENSION

Understand that some strain, some tension may have slightly sensitized you once more; or that memory, stirred by some sight, even some smell, may have flashed the old feeling again. Any one of us at times feels sensitized by strain—"on edge," apprehensive. If this happens to a person who has at one time felt panic intensely, his feeling of apprehension can so quickly flash to panic, because the way to panic in him is so well worn, that one could almost say his panic mechanism is well oiled.

MEMORY STIRS THE EMBERS

If you can accept for a long time to come—and by this I mean even years—that you can give yourself a strong flash of panic from time to time, and if you can understand that this means no more than that you are slightly sensitized for the moment, or that memory has stirred the embers of your illness, and if you can accept the panic without withdrawing from it, then you are truly recovered, despite occasional bouts of panic. *Recovery from panic always lies on the other side of panic, never on this side.*

IN SEARCH OF THE OLD SENSATIONS

You may sometimes go in search of the old sensations to try yourself out, thinking it too good to be true that you are free of the wretched things. Go ahead. You can come to no harm if you go toward them and don't withdraw from them. What cured you in the past (facing, accepting, and letting time pass) will continue to do so, in spite of any setback. So accept any setback, however long it may last, and let more time pass.

UNDERSTANDING SETBACK

The contrast between the hope and peace experienced in a good period and the renewed suffering felt in a setback highlights the setback and makes it seem more unendurable than ever. It is this contrast that may make the early setbacks seem so especially severe and brings such disappointment and despair that the sufferer may decide that the struggle to climb up the ladder to recovery again is beyond him. It seems as if some "thing" is always ready to drag him back whenever he tries to go forward.

THE WORST SETBACK OF ALL

He had thought that as he recovered, setbacks, if they occurred at all, would be less and less severe, occur less and less often. And so they might. But, as I have just explained, they may just as well seem worse than ever. Indeed, the worst setback of all may come *just before complete recovery,* just because recovery is so close. The closeness of recovery makes any setback at that time especially frustrating. And yet, however severe setback may be and however close to recovery it may come, it makes no difference to complete recovery if it is coped with the right way. That is why, when trying to recover, you should understand the tricks memory can play and understand setback so well that you are not discouraged by it, however long it may last or whenever it may come.

NEVER COMPLETELY OVERWHELMED AGAIN

When you understand setback, have adjusted your attitude to it, you have unmasked the bogy of "nerves" and they can never completely frighten you again. There will always be that inner core of confidence and strength to help you pass through fear. And because this confidence has been born the hard way, from *your own experience,* you will never quite lose it. You may falter but you will *never be completely overwhelmed again.*

As you lose your fear and regain confidence, you will lose interest in your sensations. You begin to forget yourself for moments and then for hours at a time. Outside interests claim you. You rejoin the world of other people. You are yourself again.

THE PATTERN OF RECOVERY

You recover then by *facing, accepting, floating, and letting time pass*. You are beginning to know this pattern by heart? I hope so. I want you to know it so thoroughly that your thoughts fly to it when in doubt or difficulty. It will never fail you if you apply it correctly.

10

Nervous Illness
Complicated by Problems,
Sorrow, Guilt, or Disgrace

The person suffering from the type of illness described
in the previous chapters had no major problem worrying him other than finding an escape from the physical
sensations caused by oversensitized nerves. However,
there are many people whose illness is caused by apparently insoluble problems, deep sorrow, harrowing
guilt, or disgrace. Physical sensations are only part of
their illness, and the sufferer is often so engrossed with
the cause of breakdown that he pays these physical
sensations scant notice until they are well established.
This type of illness is more complicated than the sim-
pler anxiety state, although the two types have much
in common and it may sometimes be impossible to
draw a sharp line between.

PROBLEM

An apparently insoluble problem with the conflicts
it may bring is one of the commonest causes of complicated nervous illness. A problem serious enough to start
an illness will make the sufferer recoil when he thinks
about it. Sometimes the very fineness of his sensibilities,
his very regard for honor, or his feeling of obligation
and duty prevent him from making a compromise that

another less scrupulous person would make. Most of us with a distressing problem shrink from it at first, but we eventually solve it or compromise, if necessary. The person in danger of illness dwells more and more on the unbearable aspects of the problem and finds no solution.

Whatever the problem, if it is grave enough to cause illness it will alarm the sufferer, so that from time to time, when he thinks of it, he panics. After a while he begins to feel the physical strain of continuous fear and tension and his hands sweat, he feels nauseated, his heart pounds. At first these feelings come mainly when he thinks of his problem or of anything related to it, so that the problem gradually becomes intolerable, accompanied as it is by such upsetting physical feelings.

HIS HEART SINKS LIKE LEAD

His day becomes colored by his "tragedy." He may forget it for a few moments and be happy, only to remember it suddenly in the midst of happiness, and his heart sinks like lead. He feels like a drowning man who, every time he comes up for air, is sucked under water again. He may continue for weeks, even months, like this, trying to work but gradually losing all joy in living. Eventually his work suffers. His appearance suffers and his fellow workers notice his strangeness.

This process may be gradual. However, he may go downhill quickly, holding his problem before his eyes all day and having one spasm of panic after another. Whether the downhill course be slow or quick, the pattern is much the same. The more this person dwells on his problem, the more fearful it becomes. What is more alarming, his spasms of fear become more and more intense and the slightest stimulus can start one.

The sufferer becomes bewildered. He cannot understand what has happened, and his bewilderment is increased by his vulnerability to suffering. Anything, perhaps something only remotely related to his problem, can make him panic, so he is afraid even to glance at a newspaper.

EXAGGERATED REACTION TO STRESS

Not only is he vulnerable to the fears that his problem inspires, but his reaction to any stress becomes more and more exaggerated, adding to his bewilderment. The stress of waiting is unendurable. It seems as if his brain will snap. The stress of worry becomes a real pain in his head, more than just a headache. It is a searing, pressing, hard pain that nothing seems to relieve. If obliged to do something he dislikes he may be swept by such a storm of painful emotional protest that he stands paralyzed before it. And how vulnerable he is to other people's suffering! A sight that we would think merely sad, to him seems tragic. Ordinary events become charged with unnerving poignancy. Most of us are more easily upset when tired: if we magnify this many times, we get a glimmering of the suffering experienced in such illness and can appreciate how bewildering this can be.

This person also becomes sensitized to his imagined unworthiness, and any guilt tucked away at the back of memory is now sure to raise its ugly head. We all have some guilt rationalized into quiescence. The nervously ill person has little hope of keeping guilt rationalized or submerged. As fast as one bogy raises its head and is vanquished, another comes along.

Such a patient brings a long list of guilty suffering that the doctor does his best to assuage, only to find a completely new list appearing at the next visit. Guilt can be hell indeed to a person with an oversensitized conscience. The guilt is rarely as great as the sufferer imagines. He has lost his ability to keep it in proportion, because his emotional reactions at the memory of it are so grossly exaggerated. His life to him may seem all guilt.

EXHAUSTION

As time passes the sufferer begins to tire. Nothing is more exhausting than continued emotional stress. At first he could survive much cogitation, even months of it, but gradually his mind and his emotions become fatigued. He has been thinking almost every minute of the day and may be having nightmares as well.

Normally we do not think continually. We may believe that we do, but we do not. Much of the time our brain acts like a receiving set, recording sounds and sights without actually thinking about them. It is in these moments that it rests.

Playing the Record

The person with the absorbing problem thinks about it more and more, until every waking moment is spent in thought and his mind rests only when asleep—and then only if peacefully asleep, which is rarely. Such continuous preoccupation with a small group of ideas has been likened to playing the same gramophone record ceaselessly. In the beginning the sufferer can work with the record playing in the background; but gradually it comes between him and his work, between him and his reading, between him and making contact with other people. It takes control of his mind. It becomes his mind. He used to be able to say, "I won't think of that for a while," and dismiss the unwanted subject with some success. Now, however hard he tries to get this thing off his mind, he cannot. The harder he fights, the more it clings. In other words, *his tired mind seems to have lost its resilience and thoughts race on automatically.*

The Groove

This ceaseless thinking is exhausting, terrifying, and bewildering enough, but a new and more alarming phenomenon arises. At least when this person used to think about his problem he could consider it from different points of view, but now, suddenly, he may find that he can see it only from the aspect that has been upsetting him during the past months. He can no longer think "around" his problem, only "of" it.

It is as if this viewpoint has worn a deep groove in his mind and his troubled thoughts are automatically channeled into it whenever he thinks of the problem. To see it from another angle seems beyond his power. As soon as he tries to think differently the old distressing picture flashes before him with such vividness and is accompanied by such intense, fearful emotion that it dismisses all other thoughts. This emotional reaction is triggered so quickly that it is almost a reflex.

Now he becomes truly alarmed. He is convinced he is going mad. It must be a frightening experience to stand helpless before one's own thoughts.

"This Is Me at Last!"

He clutches desperately at every moment when he feels normal. Sometimes, when watching television with the family, he may feel at peace and think, "Now this is *me* at last. This is fine. If I can stay like this, I'll be all right!" He clings to such moments, afraid to let them go for fear that if he loses them he will lose himself.

For a while after such an experience he may feel safe, even at peace, but because the past months have sensitized his nerves to react so intensely to anxiety, he has only to be anxious once more—which is inevitable in the circumstances—for his reactions to be as alarming as ever. They must be. His nerves are triggered to make them so. He despairs once more and tries even harder to grasp at outside familiar things to steady himself, to try to contact reality, to try to assure himself that all is well, that he is not mental. His spirits rise one minute and fall the next. One woman said she felt like a cork bobbing up and down in a stream at the mercy of every passing current.

Confused, Slow Thinking

I have mentioned the pain that descends like a tight band around the head and becomes worse with contemplation of the problem. This pain makes thinking so difficult that thought may become confused and slow.

Let me illustrate this type of breakdown by describing the illness of a middle-aged man who came for help. His doctor, in the course of a general examination, had found his blood pressure raised and had said, "You will probably die of a stroke." This was the patient's description of the conversation. The stunned man, not wishing to show too much concern, asked few questions but brooded all the way home. Instead of confiding in his wife, he continued to brood and say nothing. This man was about to undertake an important work demanding some years of dedication. Now, without warning, it hardly seemed worth while. He became lost in a sad dilemma. What was the use of starting a project with a stroke waiting for him? And yet he was already committed. He became so strained and worried that gradually, whenever he thought of dying of a stroke, the upsetting sensations mentioned above descended upon him.

HE WAS SUCH A SENSIBLE FELLOW!

When he first came to me he was in a pitiful state. I asked his doctor if he could help us both by describing just what was said at that interview. The doctor was surprised at the outcome of his words. Yes, he had mentioned a stroke, but had meant only that in years to come, when this man's time had come to die, he would probably have a stroke. The doctor found it hard to believe that the patient could so easily have misunderstood him and been so unnecessarily upset. He kept saying, "But he was such a sensible fellow!" So are we all sensible fellows when concerned with somebody else's health and troubles. It is different when it is our own and we are told bad news in a way that shocks us and leads to misunderstanding.

"I FEEL AS IF MY MIND IS FROZEN"

I explained this to the patient and thought he would get quick relief. Far from it. He came back and said, "Doctor, you will probably think I am a coward and a fool. I understand all you say, but I can't get it in here." He tapped his forehead. He continued: "It is as if my mind is frozen on the subject of stroke. I feel that if something would only crack inside my head I would get relief and be able to think the way I want to. As it is, I'm not in the race. I automatically feel horror every time I think of a stroke and I can't stop thinking about it. I have only to read something remotely connected with blood pressure to have these reactions."

He was too exhausted to rise above the conditioned exaggerated expression of his emotional and mental fatigue.

LOSS OF CONFIDENCE

At this stage in his illness the sufferer loses all confidence. A little child could lead him. The past months have been spent in "unending hesitation between two paths," so that now decision, even about small things, requires a Herculean effort which he finds impossible to sustain for longer than a few moments. To decide whether to take an umbrella can be a major problem, almost beyond his power. The umbrella will have a most exciting time, down the path one minute, back in the house the next, and then off down the path again. If only rain would come and clinch the matter!

And yet this man is constantly trying to prove that he is still master of himself and not the coward he is beginning to suspect he might be. He is constantly setting fresh tests of endurance and feels more and more obliged to show himself that he can still do "this" or "that." "I will do it," he says. "This is not going to get the better of me." He does it, but at what expense of nervous energy! Hence his efforts are short-lived and, as such, often criticized by his friends. In his oversensitized state he thinks his friends are criticizing more than they are.

TRICKS OF VISION

In addition he may complain that his sight is affected, that objects appear blurred and thrown into shadow. To remedy this he may keep blinking and screwing up his eyes. Certain objects may appear covered with a shimmering haze like that seen on a hot

asphalt road in summer; or they may move spasmodi-
cally when viewed from the corner of the eye. Bright
light may irritate and he may seek the relief of dark
glasses. His everyday glasses need constant readjustment
and it is difficult to find a satisfactory pair. This is
not surprising since his vision, related as it is to nervous
tension, may vary with each examination.

NOISE

Auditory nerves, oversensitized by fatigue, play
similar tricks. The gentle contact between spoon and
saucer may sound loud enough to make him wince,
and television in the house may nearly drive him
crazy. Even if he can tolerate the noise, his tired brain
has difficulty holding the thread of a plot for more
than a few seconds, and most of the time he has with-
drawn so much into himself that he cannot follow the
dialogue. It is as if the actor moves his mouth but
emits no sound. An unnerving sight, to say the least of
it, so he retires from the family circle and withdraws
even more within himself.

The inability to understand what is happening may
now be more alarming than the original conflict or
problem, which may have solved itself. The sufferer
will walk around the block, head down, thoughts
turned inward, searching for a way out of this nightmare. No solution is permanent; none suits him for
long.

It may be just at this stage that life presents extra
burdens, domestic trouble, financial worry, or perhaps
only minor aggravating experiences—trivial enough,
but exasperating to him.

WITHOUT THE VAN GOGH
HE WOULD HAVE HAD A CHANCE

For example, a patient was taken to the country for
a holiday. On arrival, he found hanging on the wall at
the foot of his bed a print of the picture of Van Gogh

with his ear cut off. Unfortunately he knew Van Gogh
had mutilated himself in this way during one of his
mad spells. Just to be in the same room with the picture was almost unendurable strain, yet how could he
tell his host he wanted the wretched thing removed?
How could he tell him he was terrified of going mad
himself and couldn't bear to be reminded of it every
time he went into the bedroom? This was a special
holiday to help his nerves. Without the Van Gogh he
would have had a chance, but of course it had to be
there.

A woman patient went to the seaside for a few weeks.
The first day at the beach she noticed a group of wom-
en standing at the water's edge looking aimlessly out
to sea. They were there the next day and the next.
They had such a strange out-of-this-world look about
them that she finally asked who they were, only to be
told they were the inmates of a city mental asylum
down on holiday. Of all times in the year they had to
choose this! Those women seemed to dog her footsteps
in that small village, and she said she never failed to
see the shadowy form of herself trooping along at their
rear.

The Exhausted Family

There is the added anxiety of watching the family,
one by one, become tired and exasperated. They are
feeling the strain of alternately hoping and despairing.
One of them is bound to say something further to upset the patient. One woman, who went to her husband
saying she thought she was going mad, was told, "Well,
there are plenty of places to send people who go like
that." He was the kindest of husbands, but his nerves
were so tensed by the continuous strain of trying to help
and placate his wife and not say the "wrong thing"
that he scarcely knew what he was saying. As it was,
he could hardly have done more harm had he taken
the last straw and placed it on her back himself.

THE FULL DEFEATIST TREATMENT

The sufferer thinks he has failed himself and his family by breaking down and is only too ready to give himself the full defeatist treatment at the slightest encouragement. Because this is all such a strain to bear, an otherwise good-natured person may find himself becoming bad tempered even with those he loves—especially with those he loves most—because, if they, of all people, cannot understand when he turns to them for help, he feels desperate, as if he is grasping at cotton candy for support.

WHAT CAN HE DO? WHERE CAN HE GO?

This person is now fatigued almost beyond human endurance and yet he cannot rest. Sensitized nerves bring agitation, so he feels impelled to rush about, although he can hardly drag his tired body along. How he longs to rest, yet when he does, all the devils of torture plague him. What can he do? Where can he go? His mood swings from depression to hysterical reaction. At times he may find relief in tears.

DEPRESSION

Depression is born from emotional fatigue. If depression strikes suddenly as a strong physical feeling, it can be a shattering experience, and it is hard to believe that the world is still a good place to live in and that recovery is worthwhile and possible. The sufferer rarely understands that this is but another expression of his extreme fatigue. Our moods are so much a part of us that it is difficult to regard them dispassionately. When the world seems black it is not easy to say, "It is I who am out of sorts, not the world."

The fight becomes grimmer and grimmer. Depression and apathy may rob their victim of the desire to recover. Every moment becomes a torture; even to comb his hair is an almost unendurable physical and mental effort, so he may begin to look unkempt.

It is at this stage that obsession may begin.

Obsession

Obsession is one of the most alarming manifestations of nervous illness and more than any other symptom convinces the sufferer that he must be on the way to madness. And yet it can start very simply in a fatigued person. Most of us have a mild obsession or two; for instance, the woman who, on going out, must return and check the faucets or gas jets, although she knows perfectly well she turned them all off before leaving.

Obsession that comes with nervous illness is more demanding than this and is characterized by repeated compulsive thought or action which is always distasteful, even fearful, to its victim. For example, the patient afraid of having a stroke developed the most aggravating obsession. When he stooped, the blood rushing to his face reminded him so forcibly of his blood pressure and the imagined stroke, that he invariably thought, "Stroke!" The harder he tried not to do so, the more surely he did. Sometimes he even said the word aloud. When new power switches were put into his home, he ordered them to be placed waist high so that he need not stoop.

Unwelcome Autosuggestion

Then there was the sick nurse who had babies under her care and could not pass a window in the hospital without feeling the urge to throw the baby in her arms into the street below. The list is long and no benefit will be gained by detailing it here. If you have obsessions it is necessary only that you should understand how they have come about and know how to cure them.

Most of us know the difficulty of banishing a tune from our mind when tired. A tired mind loses its resilience and an unwanted tune or thought sticks like a fly to flypaper. In other words, the obsession of a sufferer with nervous illness is caused by no more than unwelcome autosuggestion which, coming at a time when emotions are so grossly exaggerated, makes such an overpowering impression on the fatigued mind that it becomes firmly established there.

Anyone who has not experienced nervous illness may think I have painted an unnecessarily grim picture. I can assure such a reader that no part is exaggerated and that the actual experience is worse than the description. My reason for exposing every detail is simple. This book is written mainly for the person with nervous illness, or "bad nerves," and it is a revelation to him to learn that his mysterious and bewildering symptoms are no more than those of nervous illness in general and have been experienced by many before him. To him his body has been a Pandora's box of unpleasant surprises and he has lived in dread of what might appear next. When the whole box of tricks is laid out before him and he understands what he is facing, it loses much of its terror.

SHOCK TREATMENT

If the obsessed and depressed patient has not already consulted a psychiatrist, his family insists that he see one now and the treatment advised is sometimes shock treatment. The very sound of the words is frightening and yet, despite its name, it may bring quick relief. After shock treatment, the majority of patients temporarily forget their problems, do not worry so constantly about themselves and seem generally much better, except that they are forgetful of current as well as past events and may be slightly confused.

We do not understand how shock treatment works, but we do know that, by helping the sufferer to forget himself and his problems, it breaks the worry-tension-worry cycle. For example, a woman who had been constantly complaining about the churning in her stomach, after a few shock treatments said to her doctor, "I have a funny sort of feeling in my stomach. It is nothing to worry about, but I thought I should tell you in case the shock treatment is causing it." She had forgotten that she had continually bewailed that very feeling for weeks before and had said, only a few weeks earlier, that it was almost unendurable.

CURE YOURSELF WITHOUT SHOCK TREATMENT

My main object in writing this book is to teach you how to cure yourself *without shock treatment,* and I wish to do so for the following reasons:

1. When a person is cured by shock treatment he does not understand how the cure has come about. Therefore, were he to have a similar illness in the future, he may be no more capable of extricating himself then than now and would possibly need further shock treatment. We are all vulnerable to something we dread, and some people who have had shock treatment dread the thought of another illness and more such treatment. Living with dread, however neatly tucked away at the back of memory, does not encourage relaxation. Such a person has underlying tension, which does not portend well for overcoming future difficulties. Also, a sufferer who has had shock treatment sooner or later meets some busybody who "knows all about shock treatment" and who does not fail to inform his reluctant audience that "Once you've had shock treatment you'll always have to have it." This remark, although far from true, falls on receptive ears, because the patient already has this suspicion. Many people who have had shock treatment wish, deep in their hearts, that they could have recovered without it. They realize that if they had done so they would have been made aware of the various phases of recovery from nervous illness and so would know the way back to health. When a person knows the way back he loses his fear of becoming ill again. In place of apprehension he now has a confidence nothing can destroy. *He may know the way in, but he also knows the way out.*

A FINER CHARACTER

2. While curing himself, this person must face and overcome the human weaknesses in his character that

helped cause illness, so that when cured he is a finer person than before. The man or woman cured by shock treatment is indeed well once more, but has not this same sense of satisfying achievement or · self-mastery.

The person who has had shock treatment for some former illness and is now well and is reading this book will find something in it to help him. It will explain certain mysteries, should clarify the origin of his illness, and show him how he could have cured himself without the aid of shock treatment. It will also teach him how to avoid future illness and hence will help him to find the confidence he needs.

But I do wish to emphasize that if you are nervously ill and, after reading this book, make up your mind to recover without shock treatment, you can. However ill you may be, you can do it. At first it may seem difficult, but as time passes and brings small successes, confidence grows and more success comes with growing confidence.

You have probably seen yourself in part, if not in all, of this description. It is possible that you have difficulties not mentioned here, but the principle of treatment outlined in the next chapters will meet those difficulties.

11

How to Cure Nervous Illness Complicated by Problems, Sorrow, Guilt, or Disgrace

Although nervous illness caused by problems, sorrow,
guilt, or disgrace usually brings a very harassed sufferer with complicated symptoms to the doctor, the
same fundamental plan of treatment just described for
the more straightforward type of nervous illness cures
them, namely:

> Facing
> Accepting
> Floating
> Letting time pass

Each of the main causes of illness—problems, sorrow, guilt, and disgrace and their side effects, such as
loss of confidence, feelings of unreality, obsession, depression, etc.—will be discussed in a separate chapter.

Before studying treatment, the four following conditions for cure should be read and a resolution made to
obey them.

1. Carry out instructions wholeheartedly. A half-
hearted try is useless.

2. Never be completely discouraged by apparent
failure. However severely you may seem to fail on
occasions, *failure is only as severe as you will let it*

be. The decision to accept and carry on despite failure turns the worst failure into success. There is no "point of no return" in nervous illness. A day of deep despair can be followed by a day of hope, and just when you think you are at your worst you can turn the corner to recovery. Your emotions are so variable in nervous illness, try not to be too impressed by your unhappy moods, and never be completely discouraged.

3. There must be no self-pity. And this means *no self-pity*. There must be no dramatization of self in this "terrible state"—no thinking of how little the family understands, how little they realize how ghastly this suffering is. Self-pity wastes strength and time and frightens away those who would otherwise help you. If you are honest with yourself you will admit that some of your self-pity is pride: pride that you have withstood so much for so long. Of this you can be justly proud, and let recognition of this endurance give you confidence when you approach this new method of treatment. When I mention self-pity to some patients they look at me blankly. It had not occurred to them to pity themselves, so busy were they being bewildered. But others know exactly what I mean.

4. There must be no regretting and sighing "If only . . ." What has happened, if it cannot be remedied, is now past, finished. The present and the future must be your main concern. Life lies ahead. So remember, no more If onlys. A man came for help whose sad story was so full of "If only" that his nails were bitten down almost to the quick. However hard I tried to convince him that he should now cease regretting, accept the past, and plan for the future, he continued to return saying, "Now, if only . . ." In vain I tried to make him understand that he must find occupation to help himself regain stability. He kept saying he was too exhausted to work and far too preoccupied with his problems. His main problem was desertion by his wife. She had left him and gone to the country. During the time I treated him she came to town and inquired if he was working yet. It is possible that had the answer been "Yes" she would have returned to him. As it was,

she went back to the country. The next day he came to me saying, "Doctor, you remember telling me to get a job? Well, I'm sure that if I'd had one my wife would have come back. Now, if only I'd listened . . ." He was off again. Surely there is no need to say more to convince you that your path must lie ahead. You will often regret and often think "If only . . ."—that is human, but do not let regret hinder recovery.

> Carry out instructions wholeheartedly.
> Never be completely discouraged by failure.
> Have no self-pity.
> Let there be few regrets and fewer If onlys.

12

Problems

If some distressing problem has brought you to a state of great emotional and mental fatigue, you have probably realized that you now have little hope of making lasting decisions about your problem without help. You will certainly try to force yourself to do so, at great expense of nervous energy, but you will probably be unable to hold any decision for long and will make new, even momentous, decisions every little while. One moment you will think you have everything straightened out and feel happy about it. And then you find, perhaps only a few moments later, some new aspects of the problem that send you immediately off into indecision again.

You Seem to be Propelled

It may be a hardship to think at all. You may be so slowed by fatigue that you grope for thoughts, or your thoughts may have reached the stage where they consistently turn into the same distressing groove and deliberation over your problem seems impossible. You seem to be propelled into always thinking the same thoughts. In this condition it is essential that you seek help. You must have someone with whom to discuss your troubles and help you find a satisfactory way of looking at them. Only then will your sensitized body begin to find peace, your tired mind find rest.

It May Not Depend Entirely on You

It is as if you must temporarily use your helper's mind as your own until your mind recovers from its fatigue. This is an excellent example of how untrue are the well-worn complacent sayings, "It all depends on you," and "Your recovery is in your hands—it's up to you." Your recovery may not rest only in your own hands. You most certainly may need help.

When I explained this to a harassed woman recently she burst into tears and said, "Please don't take any notice of my tears. I'm so relieved to hear you say I need help. I feel too utterly spent to help myself much and yet everyone insists that it depends entirely on me, that no one can really help me but myself. I have been so overwhelmed and helpless at the thought of this that to hear you say I need help is almost too much to bear!"

Do not feel ashamed or discouraged if you feel you need help. An injured leg may need a crutch, why not a tired mind? But choose your helper as carefully as you can. Let it be a wise person. Do not choose a friend just because he happens to be near.

Temptation to Choose the Nearest Confidant

You are now so impressionable that the wrong advice could be upsetting and could temporarily hinder recovery. It is a temptation to choose the nearest confidant. You may have noticed how readily you confide in a stranger. As one woman expressed it, "To my shame, I find myself baring my soul to the tradesmen and I don't seem able to do much about it." Try not to talk to many and so confuse yourself with different opinions. Choose one wise friend and keep to him.

If you have no such friend, find a suitable doctor, minister, or priest. If you choose a religious confidant, be sure he is not one who will think it his duty to make you more aware of your guilt. You are probably too much aware of this already and too willing to castigate yourself, with dire results. At this stage you need comfort, not chastisement.

ACCEPT THE NEW POINT OF VIEW

After suitable deliberation with a well-chosen adviser you must be prepared to accept, for the time being at least, the solution or compromise you both find. Do not expect a perfect solution. When you are well you can modify it if necessary; it will be far easier to do so then than now. But it is essential that at this stage *you end your ceaseless pondering and are given one point of view to hold in your tired mind*. The solution finally decided upon *must be acceptable to you*. There is nothing more soul searing than trying to follow blindly a pattern not acceptable to one's heart. So do not persevere with a solution that you feel, deep within yourself, is not the right one. Peace cannot be forced in this way. It is essential that the new view causes a minimum of pain and fear. A wise counselor will see to this. Ask him first to read this book, so that he will understand the part expected of him.

YOU MAY NOT FIND A POINT OF VIEW ENTIRELY WITHOUT PAIN

Talking about the new point of view will help to impress it on your mind. Also, ask your friend to write it down as simply as possible, so that you can refer to it when alone. I repeat, *holding one point of view will act as a crutch for your tired mind*. It delivers you from ceaseless cogitation and its resulting emotional and mental fatigue. You may not find a viewpoint entirely without pain, but knowing it is the best available brings some peace, some respite.

To discuss your problem with another may mean forcing yourself to expose something, the mere thought of which brings on such paroxysms of fear that you may think you are incapable of dragging yourself to your friend. Do not make the mistake of forcing yourself to go, of fighting your way there. You will arrive exhausted if you do. Use the pattern of recovery described earlier and *float there*. Do you remember the woman who could not enter a shop until she learned the trick of floating? Follow her example and imagine you are floating. It works like magic. As I have explained, when you think of floating you automatically relax a little, and this lessens tension which has been inhibiting action. So "float" to your friend, don't fight your way there. In addition, try, as I mentioned earlier, to release all disturbing, obstructive thoughts. Such thoughts cling, and releasing them may call for real effort, but you can succeed with practice.

THE IRON BAND

It is possible that at this stage the mere thought of talking about, or even thinking of, your problem will cause your scalp muscles to spasm and bring the iron band of pain around your head. Do not be dismayed by this. You can still think, *if you are prepared to accept the pain and relax your head muscles to the best of your ability.* You may be forced to think slowly, and because of this may feel confused. Accept the slow thought and confusion without panic. Do not fight it by tensing your muscles and trying to force thought. If you relax with acceptance you will find that you can still think adequately, however slowly. *There is nothing wrong with your brain; its work is only being hindered by pain, fear, and fatigue. Its eventual recovery will be complete.*

OLD FEARS RETURN

While you are discussing your problem with your confidant you may feel overwhelming relief and think you are cured at last. This may be true, especially if you have not had such help before. This person may give you such healing comfort and such a satisfactory solution to your problem that you may have no more suffering. Also, confession alone can cure, if your troubles called for confession.

However, if you have suffered for months and have already experienced discussion and confession, although you may feel immediate relief when you discuss your problems again, the relief may be temporary. Your nerves are still fatigued and so may yet play tricks on you. You may think you have straightened out your problem with your adviser, only to find, when you are alone again, that some hitherto unsuspected and undiscussed aspect presents itself, and once more alarming, exaggerated reactions throw you into panic.

Or you may find that, while able to follow your friend's reasoning when with him, and able to hold it for some time after leaving him, your old fears eventually return and you lose your grip on the new point of view. Do not despair at this. It is to be expected. After all, you have been looking at the problem for so long from the one distressing viewpoint that it would be almost a miracle if this did not soon reassert itself vividly. It has become your habit pattern.

So if you find that the old point of view returns with all its upsetting accompaniments, go once more to your friend, tell him about it, and discuss your problem again. Indeed, you may have to visit him often before you can grasp and hold firmly the new point of view. A wise counselor must also be very patient.

A HINDRANCE INTO A HELP

As mentioned, it is a great help if your adviser writes down a few notes for you. I make such notes or tape recordings for my patients and, if necessary, with the patient's consent, show a member of his family how to help him. I sometimes coach the very member who has been most unsympathetic and who may have been making the patient's life even more of a burden. In this way I have turned a hindrance into a help. It is surprising how enthusiastic such people can become when they think they have the doctor's confidence and that he is turning to them for co-operation. From being critical of the doctor they uphold his opinion as if it were the final appeal.

GLIMPSING THE NEW POINT OF VIEW

If after obtaining the help of your friend, or perhaps some member of your family, you find that you can hold the new viewpoint for only a few moments each day, do not be discouraged. *If you can just glimpse it for a fleeting moment daily you will have made a beginning.* Eventually, with practice, you will be able to glimpse more readily and hold that glimpse longer and longer, until you make it the final established point of view. Then you will be at peace.

THE FARMER'S WIFE

Let me illustrate this with a story about a farmer's wife. She had lived happily with her husband and children on a small farm with good friends nearby until she became ill with pneumonia. During her convalescence the children were sent to boarding school and the friends moved farther into the country, so that this woman was left lonely and unemployed when she most needed company and occupation. Days spent on the farm became a misery.

Had she realized at this stage that her troubles were the expression of exhaustion following pneumonia, she would have been saved much additional suffering. As it was, she became bewildered and afraid of her condition and, on the advice of a friend, visited a psychoanalyst. She made an unfortunate choice, was inexpertly analyzed, and an odd collection of small, pathetic guilt complexes was exposed as it would be in any one of us similarly treated. The analyst made much of this guilt and of course, with his encouragement, so did the patient, so that she now found herself with a bunch of problems to solve. She became more apprehensive and depressed and developed a protracted nervous illness.

I SEEM TO BE A DIFFERENT PERSON

She could not understand why the home she had loved and where she had been so happy could upset her now so that she could hardly bear to think about it. She did not wish her husband to be obliged to sell at that time because this would have been financially unwise. She said, "I just want to live happily at home, but this seems utterly beyond my power. What has happened to me? I seem to be a different person." She said that as soon as she drew near the place a wave of such deep revulsion swept over her that she wanted to run away.

I explained to her that she was looking at the situation from two conflicting points of view. First, she saw the farm as a place where she had recently suffered deep depression, and the memory was so vivid and frightening that she was convinced that the same suffering, or worse, was waiting to claim her again as soon as she entered the house. Second, and at the same time, she saw her home as the place where she had lived happily in the past and where she wanted to do so again.

I explained that she must put before herself the picture of living contentedly there and must be prepared to wait for time to pass until this picture became reality. *It would take time for the memory of her suffering to fade.* Until it did, she could not expect much happiness there. She might have happy moments, but *only time could establish happiness by fading the memory of unhappiness.*

In the meantime she must be occupied and let each day pass *without watching her own reactions and analyzing her feelings.* The feelings of the present and the immediate future were sure to be mixed, uncertain, and painful, colored as strongly as they were by the recent past, so why be impressed by them? She must be prepared to live through the next few months while she gradually floated toward her goal. *Wanting to live at home happily was enough foundation to build on.* I explained that by "float" I meant she must let time carry her to happiness and must not ask for quick recovery.

As it is not wise for depressed people to be alone for long, I advised this woman to make frequent visits into town and to invite a friend to stay with her while waiting for the new point of view to become established. It is inestimable help to a patient with a nervous illness just to hear another person moving about the house.

STICK TO THE NEW POINT OF VIEW

If you too wish to forget an upsetting point of view, do so by finding a more acceptable substitute, and when you have found one, *stick to it*. If changed circumstances make readjustment necessary, consult your adviser, unless you are so much better that you are certain you can manage unaided. If you have any doubts about yourself you must seek help again, otherwise you will be caught in the same old habit of thinking one way one moment and another the next.

It is not necessary to make your own decisions at this stage. You gain no lasting benefit by trying to do so. Above all, *do not waste time being upset because you cannot make decisions*. Realize you are like this because of fatigue and that as soon as you are well again you will be as capable as ever of making up your own mind, perhaps after this experience more capable. I emphasize, it is not important that you make decisions now. It is important only that you and your adviser arrive at one decision about your problem and that you abide by it and so rest your tired brain.

A man who complained of being unable to make decisions was told that he had but to make a supreme effort and reach a decision and his battle would be won. From then on, added his adviser, he would have no more trouble making decisions.

This advice was misleading. This person may make a great effort and successfully arrive at one decision, but that will not alter the fact that his mind still seems non-resilient and his nerves are still sensitized, so that in the immediate future it could be just as difficult as ever for him to make decisions. Why place so much importance on the necessity for a tired mind to make decisions? When the mind rests with relief from fear, decisions will be more easily made.

THE INSOLUBLE PROBLEM

On being advised to find a solution or a compromise to their problem, some people think, "My problem has no solution, so there's no way out for me." I have seen too many apparently insoluble problems solved to be impressed by this. Your problem may seem insoluble to you, but you would be surprised at what an experienced counselor can unravel. If little can be done to alter a situation, at least he can teach you to look at it from a less distressing point of view. For example, a woman made ill by living with a mother-in-law of whom it was impossible to be rid said "So, you see, Doctor, there is no solution for me."

I explained that there was no solution while she regarded her mother-in-law's absence as the only way out of the difficulty. I suggested that instead of looking at the old woman with hate, she should make a determined effort to concentrate on her good points and see if she could feel differently toward her. People react to our opinion of them and very often act toward us as they subconsciously think we expect them to. The old woman must have known of her daughter-in-law's dislike and probably, as a result, unwittingly turned her worst side toward the girl. Happily the young woman came to understand this and was successful in changing the situation.

TRUE ORGANIC SICKNESS

It is not easy to be philosophical about ill health based on organic sickness that is not "just nerves." If such illness is the cause of your nervous illness, you need aid from an understanding doctor because, even here, there may be a medical point of view that can help you.

For many years an old friend of mine, now aged eighty-five, has had persistently high blood pressure. Fifteen years ago, when she first knew about the pressure, she was about to succumb to the fear of an imagined imminent stroke. However, after a few quiet talks her doctor was able to help her view the situation sensibly. How fortunate that he did, otherwise this woman could have spent the last fifteen years of her life fearfully awaiting a stroke that has not come.

CHANGE OF SCENE

In nervous illness there may be the stultifying repetition of the same old familiar scene and a daily encounter with painful memories associated with it. Many a person craves change and feels that he should not be battling against such odds as these. However, his friends so often advise him to "stick to his guns," that he stays, thinking that to flee the scene would be considered cowardly.

A situation should be carefully considered before advising anyone to stay on the scene of nervous illness. If leaving would be running away from something that should be faced, then I recommend staying. However, even here it is often wise to leave temporarily until more rested. For example, a young schoolteacher came to me with a nervous illness caused by failing to control a class of unruly pupils. I did not advise this woman to quit and find a different school. Had she done so, she may have met another unruly class or at least would have always lived in dread of doing so. I advised her to have a month's holiday and then return and face the class with a new method of approach. She was successful in time and very pleased that she had not changed schools.

WOUNDS OPENED DAILY HEAL TOO SLOWLY

But when a man suffering from nervous illness because his wife had left him came for help I advised him to leave the home charged with her memory until he had developed some immunity to suffering, or, better still, to leave town for six months if possible. Wounds that are opened daily heal too slowly.

So the circumstances of each person must be assessed before recommending complete change of scene. However, short changes are good for all and are often advocated. They act as mild shocks, relieve the fatigue engendered by repetition, and so help the sufferer to see himself and his problem in better perspective.

A young man suffering from nervous illness visited an unfamiliar seaside resort with friends. On entering the hotel lounge he noticed a cheerful group of people talking by a sunny window and an unusual small carved model of an old sailing ship suspended from the rafters. That glimpse of interesting difference arrested his racing thoughts, drew him out of himself, and he suddenly had insight into his strange condition. For the first time he realized that he was emotionally spent and that because of this he had his problems completely out of proportion. They were not as insuperable as he had imagined. He saw that were he well he could probably cope with them.

THE STRAIN OF SIMPLY
WAITING FOR SOMEONE TO RETURN

This young man described how, late that same evening, tense and distraught, he waited for his friends to return from a swim. The strain of simply waiting for someone to return so that he could settle for the night was almost intolerable. He felt his brain would snap. This, following on the incident in the lounge, showed him even more clearly that the trouble lay within himself, in his own exhausted physical state, and not in his problems.

Some people in a similarly spent condition complain that they feel as though they are groping beneath a low, flat, dark, unyielding ceiling that seems to press them down whenever they try to rise above their problems and think clearly. Others describe their mind as feeling as if enveloped in a gray blanket from whose folds it cannot free itself. When one remembers that eyesight may also be affected so that landscape may appear thrown into shadow even on a bright day, one can appreciate how easily these people may develop a feeling of withdrawal from the rest of the world.

CANNOT PACK IN ANOTHER WORD

This gray ceiling, or blanket, is no more than accentuated brainfag. Students experience something of this when, after three or four hours of continuous study, they suddenly feel they cannot pack in another word and must go outside and hose the garden until their mind clears. The person with nervous illness has been studying his problem for weeks, months without hosing his garden. It is not strange that his mind should feel gray, unresponsive, non-resilient, and so very, very tired.

It is not unusual to find these people craving to be on top of a high mountain or in an airplane where, they imagine, the feeling of looking down on the world below would free them from this imprisoned feeling of being under everything. This person really needs sleep, days and nights of it; sleep, and the rest that it brings from ceaseless, anxious thinking.

THE CURTAIN LIFTS

As the sufferer recovers, the curtain lifts from time to time and he has moments of joy when he can think freely and direct his thoughts with his old accustomed agility. The first moment of facile thinking may come almost as a revelation. The young man described above said that a few days after he returned from the seaside a friend asked him to bandage a cut finger. Suddenly, during the "operation," the curtain lifted and he almost shouted, "I can think clearly again!"

This man was intelligent and was able to trace the cause of his symptoms and treat himself, asking for little help. He described how, after that experience when bandaging the finger, the curtain soon descended again, to lift a few hours later. During the next few days it would lift one minute and descend the next, so that he could never be sure of himself. It was as if his mind were fragile and he must handle it with care lest it should break. He felt himself growing tense, trying to steady his mind and keep the curtain from descending. Then he remembered my words about accepting and floating, and he relaxed and accepted the hovering curtain and waited for more time to pass.

Some friends in a distant state asked him to visit them, and he knew that were he to go, the complete and sudden change would be so refreshing that the curtain would lift permanently and he would step right out of illness. He preferred to stay and prove to himself that he could recover on his own ground without outside help. When he finally was freed he said it was as if he had been reborn. Everything now shone as never before. Colors were brighter, more vivid; the blue of the sky seemed exquisite, and a feeling of such happiness and benevolence toward all things welled up within him that he could not bear to hurt even an ant. He has never completely lost that feeling. If you are suffering as this young man, the same reward awaits you. The law of compensation works particularly well after recovery from nervous illness.

This does not mean that you should refuse a change of scene if offered it. You need not prove anything to yourself. You can take this young man's word that it is possible to come out of nervous illness on your own ground without going away. But if you have suffered, why prolong it? The opportunity of having a complete change should be grasped and the relief that it can bring accepted.

RECOVERY

Recovery, then, from nervous illness caused by some apparently insoluble problem lies, first, in understanding and losing fear of the bodily symptoms that accompany the stress of long anxious brooding and, second, in learning how to compromise by finding, if not a perfect solution, as least a satisfactory way of looking at the problem. It lies in then practicing glimpsing this new point of view until it is established as the final point of view. Glimpsing may be difficult

at first, but it is a most important part of treatment.
So:

Discuss your problem with a wise counselor until
you find a satisfactory solution or compromise;
search for a second picture.

Stick to the new point of view, and be contented if
at first you can only glimpse it each day.

Remember that having one approach to your problem acts like a splint for a tired mind.

If fatigue makes concentration difficult, do not tensely try to force thought; be prepared to think as
slowly as your tired brain allows.

Do not despair if old fears return; accept all setbacks and float on to recovery.

Do not place importance on making your own decisions while ill.

Accept a change of scene if it is offered.

13

Sorrow

Although overwhelming sorrow can temporarily disorganize our lives, it is not so complicated to manage as apparently insoluble problems. Sorrow may bring problems, it is true, but these are usually overshadowed by the grief itself. Deep sorrow alone can cause nervous illness without the addition of conflict or guilt. However, when the source of such an illness is studied, it is usual to find fear somewhere involved. As mentioned earlier, sorrow at the loss of a loved one is mixed with the fear of facing the future alone.

BROODING

Many of us, when we suffer deeply, may think we are overwhelmed; however, as time passes, life carries us with it and we rally and find happiness. But there are people who become so affected by sorrow, and whose environment offers such little encouragement, that they find it impossible to lead a normal existence. They sit and think only of their ill fate. This continuous melancholic brooding gradually exhausts their emotional reserves, so that their reactions become exaggerated, their sadness becomes deeper and deeper, the waves of despair more and more overwhelming, and the body subjected to this assault becomes less and less able to withstand it.

These people eat and sleep little and literally fade away. Finally the mind becomes so exhausted, it perceives and thinks so slowly that it seems impossible to communicate with them. They stare vacantly and answer hesitatingly, if at all. If the doctor cannot penetrate this unresponsiveness, shock treatment is usually advised, and the result may be so good that after a few treatments the patient can discuss the future rationally and with hope.

An Italian woman was brought to me by her despairing family. Her husband had died six months earlier and she had become so slowed down by grief that she followed her daughter wherever she went, like a child, in a lifeless, mechanical way. When I spoke to her she merely looked blankly. As my words were making no impression, I advised shock treatment.

After a month in a hospital her one wish was to get home as quickly as possible and help with the grape picking. This woman stands as an excellent example of the blessings of shock treatment in such circumstances. It shows how, if the chain of sorrow-brooding-sorrow can be broken, the sufferer is capable of accepting life again.

THE SUFFERING HABIT

It is possible that this woman could have recovered without shock treatment, had she had help earlier and been shown where she was drifting. So much of our suffering is due to memory and habit. We remember what we suffered yesterday and fail to appreciate the difference between reality and memory. This woman's husband had been dead six months; no grieving could bring him back; she lived in a large farmhouse with a family who needed her care. That was reality, and after shock treatment she recognized it. And yet before treatment she spent her time brooding over the memory of the past until nothing but that existed, and that certainly was not reality.

Suffering soon brings fatigue, which brings more fatigue, because we grow so tired of feeling tired. However, let us bring even a little hope into our destructive thinking and we can begin to reverse the process. Hope with its forward projection also becomes memory, but an uplifting one. If we were hopeful yesterday, we can be a little more so today and even more so tomorrow, until all our days bring hope. If we are fortunate, circumstances force concentration on other things. A mother with children to care for usually recovers sooner from the death of her husband than a childless widow.

It is surprising how, even after much sorrow, we can be happy again as time passes. A woman who had had more sorrow than it would seem possible to live with, and who had lost all desire to live, said that one day, when feeling almost completely overwhelmed, she made herself go outside and burn up some garden refuse. By chance she threw some fresh leaves onto the fire. The pungent smell of burning leaves gave her a moment of unexpected pleasure, and at the same time a cheeky little bird flashed past and cavorted on a branch beside her. She could not help smiling. This experience was the turning point in her illness. It showed her that she was still capable of feeling pleasure; that such feeling was not quite as dead as she had thought. This gave her enough hope to cling to, and she now lives as peacefully and happily as most of us.

AVOID UNNECESSARY SUFFERING

If you find living with your dead husband's armchair upsets you, put it away until you can look at it with less suffering. A friend of mine refused to remove her husband's chair, saying, "I loved him when alive, why should I now avoid things that remind me of him?" While praiseworthy, this was a waste of emotional effort. For months, every time she passed the chair she suffered. She would sometimes feel moderately cheerful until she saw the chair. In the end she let us remove it temporarily. Had she done so earlier, she would have been saved unnecessary suffering. It would have been sensible, not cowardly, as she had thought. It is sometimes good to know when to run away from suffering. The backwaters of memory can make a good burial ground, and it is not wise to dig there unnecessarily.

DESERTION

While death causes sorrow, at least there is no great conflict attached to it. It is final and we must accept it. Time will help us now. Sorrow that is being constantly revived, as occurs in desertion by wife or husband, is much harder to bear. The one hears about the other, and salt is repeatedly rubbed into the wound. Injustice may be involved and this is hard to accept. But, even here, the years gradually change sorrow into acceptance and forgetfulness. One woman was very close to nervous illness after her husband left her. Now, five years later, she would not change the pattern of her life to take him back. And yet, when he went I could never have convinced her that in such a short time she would prefer his absence.

It is well to remember that *none of us depends entirely on another for our happiness,* although we may think we do. It is not the person we love who is responsible for our depth of feeling. This feeling is part of ourselves, is our capacity to love, and it stays with us despite misfortune.

So, should the person you love have left you, do not think the end of the world has come. You still have a great capacity for loving and it is possible to love someone else as much, perhaps even more, although you may shrink indignantly from this suggestion today. *Let time pass and do not hesitate to put your faith in the healing power of its passing.*

BEAR NO GRUDGE

If you have been hurt, do not make the mistake of thinking you will find relief by taking revenge or watching retribution catch up with the offender. Do not burn yourself up with the desire to "get even." To find lasting peace you must forget vengeance. The Bible gives good advice about this. It is only too true that should retribution find the one who has hurt us, we rarely feel the pleasure we anticipated. We are much more likely to have ceased being interested, or may even feel sorry for the "poor devil." So don't waste time and energy being revengeful now.

When you decide to take the kindest course, it is surprising how complications that may have seemed insuperable have a knack of disappearing. Can you see how much more peaceful and wholesome such a course would be than being burned up and kept tensed by hatred, bitterness, and impatience for revenge?

Accept your sorrow philosophically.

Do not sit and brood.

Occupy your time.

Be determined to bring hope into the picture.

Temporarily remove objects that bring painful memories.

Remember that nobody's happiness depends entirely on another.

Leave vengeance to God.

14

Guilt and Disgrace

GUILT

Guilt can be a nightmare to some people suffering with nervous illness, particularly to those trying to set a high standard for themselves, such as religious people who lead a dedicated life.

GUILTY THOUGHTS

The guilt may be associated only with thoughts. Such thoughts assume undue importance to these saintly people, who struggle to banish them by fighting them, by trying not to think them. I explain to these patients that continued recurrence of these thoughts is due to no more than fear and memory working together. As such, they will cling for the time being and must be temporarily accepted. These particular thoughts have been recurring for weeks, months, or longer. They are deeply entrenched. Thinking them has become such a habit, what hope would anyone have of banishing them immediately on command? And yet how desperately some try to do just that. The only chance of obliterating them under these conditions would be to fall unconscious or into a dreamless sleep.

NOT SO GUILTY AFTER ALL

When I point this out the victim usually feels great relief because he realizes that, even though the thoughts may hold an element of reluctant enjoyment, he is not such a particularly sinful person after all, just an ordinary human being reacting in a normal way.

Understanding banishes fear for many, and with fear lost the battle is won. The unwelcome thoughts come, but they no longer mean so much, so that, by degrees, whether they are there or not no longer matters and forgetfulness eventually follows.

GUILTY ACTION

If some past guilty action is an important part of the cause of your illness, confess and make reparation if possible, but do not be disappointed if you do not immediately feel the relief expected. Your nerves are still sensitized and will probably find some new guilt in exchange for the old. Do not be impressed by this. Try to see it for what it is, no more than the unbalanced, exaggerated reaction of sensitized nerves.

While guilt alone can start nervous illness, it is more usual for a guilt complex to arise in the course of an already established illness. Emotions, sensitized by prolonged stress, respond so quickly to some real or imagined guilt that the sufferer may find himself grappling with one guilty episode after another.

So when you have unburdened yourself of your present guilt, enjoy your relief while you may. It may be lasting, but do not be disappointed if it is not. When cured, you will feel your guilt so much less acutely that you will be able to consider it rationally and keep it in proportion.

GUILT THAT CANNOT
BE CONFESSED AND FORGIVEN

Religious people can repent in prayer or at confession, so that even if they have harmed someone now dead, they can find solace. If you are in a similar situation but can find no help in religion, face the facts squarely and decide to make amends in some way. Do not force yourself to do this immediately if the strain seems too great. It is enough to decide now to make amends later. I emphasize this aspect of not forcing, because one of the principles of treatment is to give yourself as little extra strain as possible while ill. You and your adviser must judge how important to your recovery are immediate confession and reparation and act accordingly.

We all have countless ancestors whose frailties we are bound to have inherited in some measure. Few of us can reach middle age without some skeleton rattling in our cupboard. In fact, most of us have a fine collection hidden away, but we wisely manage to lose the key. To let past guilt paralyze present action is destructive living. Let us recognize our guilt if it declares itself, make what reparation we can, but with a quiet determination live on, philosophically laying some of the blame at the feet of our ancestors, some at the feet of those who trained or neglected to train us, and some at our own feet. But let us make amends by leading from now on (in your case when you are well) worthwhile, constructive lives.

Another Chance

It would soon be an empty world if the guilty ones decided they could not live on because of their guilt. How much more commendable it is to live on cheerfully, accepting the burden of guilt. This in itself is part penance. So, *always give yourself the benefit of another chance. You can never fall so far that you cannot rise again and be a fine person,* if you make up your mind to do so. The farther the fall, the steeper the climb and the greater the effort needed for recovery, admittedly, but the character of the person who finally emerges triumphant is much finer for that extra effort.

Such endeavor does not mean gritting your teeth and fighting an uphill battle, constantly reminding yourself of your objective. It simply means putting before you the picture of the person you want to be and letting time carry you to its realization. This picture will materialize more easily if, each morning before rising, you take the time to think about it. You need make no further conscious effort to remember it during the day. You strengthen your subconscious with a daily reminder that helps to condition your actions until practice establishes the habit you seek. There is no grim battle to fight. Harness your subconscious, direct its powerful machinations with a daily reminder, and let it work a miracle for you. It can.

But remember, you must never be completely discouraged by failure. Sometimes you will think you have lost sight of your goal, but if you want it again *it will always be there.* Desire shapes your actions, therefore remember that while you have the desire you have the main requisite for success.

DISGRACE

We feel guilt because of our own actions, but we can feel disgrace because of the actions of others. A colleague of mine described how she watched her charwoman grow more and more haggard after her son had been sent to prison. Trying to comfort the old woman, she said, "Don't worry. The time will soon pass and he will be out again." She received the answer, "It's not that, Doctor, it's the disgrace."

It is not easy to comfort people made ill by such disgrace. We can tell them how passing time dulls people's memories; how a mantle of disgrace is ready for each of us if we care to wear it; how reparation and repentance can even the score. We can point out that our feeling is no more than a mixture of hurt pride and fear of public opinion, and that if we can rise above this and think of the feelings of the one who has disgraced us and who may be suffering far more than we, we shall have done a fine thing. We can do all this and find that the disgrace is still hard to bear.

If you are ill because of such disgrace, you have the compassion, not the censure, of every humane person. Also, those who love you will love you more, not less, because of your disgrace.

If your own actions have disgraced you, you have

no alternative but to study where you failed and be
determined not to do so again. And remember that
most people like to see a disgraced person make
good. It restores their faith in human nature, maybe
even in themselves. A few idle tongues will wag a little
more than usual, but their prattle is worthless at any
time. Concentrate on your true friends. Take the encouragement they offer.

15

Simple Explanation of Strange Experiences in Nervous Illness

While problems, sorrow, guilt, or disgrace can start or play an important part in nervous illness, the side effects of the continuous state of fear they may produce may bring some very strange experiences, and these may gradually take precedence over the original cause of the illness. The most usual experiences are:

Indecision, suggestibility, loss of confidence, feelings of personality disintegration, feelings of unreality, obsession, depression.

These experiences develop very much in the order in which I have just stated them. That is the pattern. In the following chapters I will show how each experience develops, how easily one leads to the other and how each depends on sensitization through stress. There is no mystery here, no need for bewilderment.

INDECISION, SUGGESTIBILITY, LOSS OF CONFIDENCE

First comes indecision. I have already mentioned how indecision often accompanies sensitization. Intense feeling follows the slightest anxious thought so swiftly that the sensitized person seems to be at the mercy of his feelings as if they are beyond his control. He has but to think on one aspect of a problem to feel immediately a strong emotional reaction to it; and then he has only to think about a different aspect to feel just as strongly about it. These swiftly changing reactions interfere with calm, clear thinking and so make deciding seem almost impossible. The nervously ill person thinks one way one minute, and another the next. Each point of view seems equally important, equally right, and yet, a moment later, equally wrong. As I said earlier, even the simple decision to take an umbrella may seem beyond him.

PITIFULLY SUGGESTIBLE
TO HIS OWN DESTRUCTIVE SUGGESTIONS

Because a nervously ill person finds difficulty in making up his own mind, he is vulnerable to suggestions of others. He may be pitifully suggestible to his own destructive suggestion that he will never recover. His reaction to this may be terrific.

THE PATTERN UNFOLDS

Because of indecision and suggestibility, loss of confidence must inevitably follow. How could it not? Can you see how the pattern unfolds? Such a logical pattern when we understand how exaggerated emotions can delude us.

FEELINGS OF
PERSONALITY DISINTEGRATION

Many nervously ill people say they feel their loss of confidence so acutely it is as if their personality has disintegrated. Because his emotional reactions are so unpredictable, so exaggerated, so frightening, and come so quickly, the sufferer feels no inner strength on which to depend, no inner self from which to seek direction. It is this lack of inner harmony holding thought and feeling together that leads him to choose the word "disintegration" to describe the way he feels.

Old-fashioned sayings can be surprisingly apt when

applied to nervous illness. The saying, "Pull yourself together," describes so well what the sick person feels he should do but feels he cannot do. It is as if he must gather the scattered pieces of his personality together and fit them into place, as one would a jigsaw puzzle, before he can be himself again. To do this he usually has to overcome the human weaknesses that helped cause his illness, and he must do this *while under great stress,* so that as he recovers he is integrated on a higher plane, is a better person.

He Was Sure the Work Was Too Much for Him

A young doctor came for help. He had lost confidence after a series of domestic mishaps, and he was so tired from fear and worry that his work suffered. To give a simple injection became a battle. Each day was spent fighting such battles until he was sure the work was too much for him. He panicked and wanted to give up studying medicine. He used the term disintegration when describing his state.

I explained the cause of his apparent disintegration and emphasized that he could continue successfully if, instead of meeting each situation with tense determination to overcome it, he were to relax, accept his present condition as temporary, and float past the reactions aroused by any aspects of his work that now dismayed him. In other words, to do his best as calmly as he could and be satisfied with the results, recognizing that to expect more from himself in his present fatigued, sensitized condition would be foolish. I explained fully the meaning of "float."

On the Verge of Laying Down His Tools

The young man returned later, a different person. "I have learned the trick of floating," he said. He told me that his first experience on returning to the hospital had been grueling. He had been obliged to give an anesthetic which, in his nervous condition, had seemed particularly difficult. To make matters worse, the surgeon, scalpel in hand, had turned to him and said, "I suppose, young man, that you know this patient has a weak heart?" The young man was on the verge of laying down his tools when he recalled my words. He knew he was capable of giving the anesthetic, so he floated past the destructive suggestion that he could not do it, reminded himself that this was only a thought, released it, and quietly went on. He had no more trouble.

I do not advise all sufferers from nervous breakdown to stay at their posts, particularly at such a difficult one as this. Each person's problem must be assessed, and it is sometimes wiser to leave work temporarily.

Do not be alarmed by the term "disintegration" if you have not heard it before. Your personality has not truly disintegrated. Your adrenalin-releasing nerves are merely oversensitized by fear and continuous tension, and your mind slowed by fatigue. This creates the illusion of disintegration. When your emotional reactions calm, you will quickly feel integrated again. You are now passing through a very temporary phase. Integration and confidence return together. One depends on the other, and both depend on peace of mind.

A New Feeling Is Born

In the beginning you may not be able to follow confidently the advice given in this book, going steadfastly forward. *The most to be hoped for at first is that you decide to try to do as shown.* You will find that that decision in itself will give you a new feeling, admittedly a little shaky at first, but nevertheless a new feeling will be born. Your confidence grows and hope comes into the picture as you see the method work. The return of confidence plays a big part in determining the rate of your recovery. Remember, the power of a muscle can depend on the confidence with which it is used.

You may despair again and again. This is not important if you remember never to despair completely and are always willing to pick up the pieces and go on.

If you do this, you will one day feel the confidence you need so much. It will be born from your relaxed acceptance of all the strange sensations associated with your nervous illness and the determination never to admit defeat. When I said this to one woman she said, "How can I never admit defeat?" The answer is that you are never defeated while you are ready to go on.

Ups and Downs

The road to recovery is beset with many temporary failures. It is like traveling across the foothills toward the mountains. You travel downhill so often that it is difficult to realize that, in spite of this, you are still climbing. This up and down aspect of recovery is exhausting and frustrating. I remember one young man saying, "I'm tired of being up one minute and down the next. I'd almost rather stay down all the time and be done with it!"

It is true that just when you think you have turned the corner and are feeling well, you can have one of your worst setbacks. You can waste much energy trying to discover why this happens. A patient will say, "I had a wonderful week last week, Doctor, the best yet, and then on Saturday and Sunday I felt terrible, as bad as ever. How is this possible?"

Do Not Measure Progress Day by Day

It may have been some trivial event that drew him back, but is it so important to find out? Strangely enough, it always seems so to the sufferer. Actually, it is important only to realize that tomorrow is another day and could be the best yet, however upsetting yesterday or today may have been. Do not measure your progress day by day. *Looking forward hopefully with confidence is tremendous help. It draws you past the yesterdays, past today, past the tomorrows until you find recovery.*

The slipping-back process is easy to understand. The past holds so many fearful memories for the person who has had a nervous illness that even a slight setback will find a host of them ready to engulf him. It takes time to dull these memories; but after he has pulled himself out of a few such reverses he despairs less readily, and confidence grows from each experience. When you have achieved confidence by your own effort, nothing can take it away again. No future defeat can quite destroy it. It may seem in moments of despair that it has gone, but the memory of past successes, however small, gives you the courage to try again, and so defeat is defeated.

So, recognize that:

Disintegration is no more than bombardment by exaggerated emotional reaction accompanied by slow, confused thinking and is caused by emotional and mental fatigue.

Integration will return with peace of mind and peace of body.

Confidence is born by going on despite defeat.

In spite of ups and downs on the road to recovery, the main direction is upward.

Confidence earned from your own experience will never leave you completely.

16

A Feeling of Unreality

It is not unusual to hear a patient say "I cannot make contact with other people. It is as though they are in one world and I in another, unreal world. However hard I try, I can't find my way back into their world. Am I going mental, Doctor?" He may have this feeling of unreality in flashes, or he may think he has it always with him.

When desperately concerned with our own problems it is not easy for any one of us to be interested in a neighbor's new car. It is even more difficult for a nervously ill person, whose thoughts are constantly reverting to himself, who is so constantly anxious about himself. It is this narrowing of interest to himself that leads to a feeling of withdrawal from the outside world, a feeling as if there is a curtain between it and him, a curtain he can neither lift nor break through.

"I FEEL I'M OUTSIDE MYSELF NOTICING MYSELF"

A nervously ill person may feel unreal in many different ways. He may say "I feel I'm outside myself watching myself," or he may say, "When I touch things, I know I'm doing it, but I can't *feel* I'm doing it." Another may say, "It seems so unreal to hear somebody laughing." Laughter seems unreal because his world of introspection has been charged with such suffering that he cannot feel in tune with laughter. He has almost forgotten how to laugh.

Shocked by the Mental State He Thought He Was In

One young man described his feeling of unreality dramatically. He said that on one occasion, when going for a swim, he had to pass through a dark passageway before emerging into the full sunshine of the beach. The sudden contrast between deep shadow and brilliant sun was so arresting that it made him acutely aware of a strange feeling of isolation, almost of darkness within himself. The crowds of laughing people and gaily colored beach umbrellas, although so close, seemed miles away, as if on a stage and he merely looking on. The harder he tried to become part of the scene, the farther it seemed to recede, the more unreal it became. He was shocked by the mental state he thought he was in. Actually, brainfag from so much anxious brooding had gradually dulled his world; it was as if he had lived for months in a gray tunnel without realizing it. Small wonder that the sudden contrast of brilliant sunshine on white sand and gay colors came as a shock. This was a natural happening and not the approaching madness he thought it was. Had he not become alarmed by it and so made himself more aware of it, his feeling of unreality would have soon passed.

The Transference Must Be Gradual

The feeling of inability to be part of the world around is accentuated by impatience to step straight out of one world, the sick world, into the other. The transference can be only gradual. It may take months for a nervously ill person to become sufficiently interested in everyday life to become part of it so that it feels real.

Normal Emotions Frozen

The illusion of loss of contact with other people can be so strong that some people complain they can feel no love for those they used to love, even for their own children. It is as if they have a vacuum where their feelings should be. Such a person has merely complicated his feeling of withdrawal by exhausting his capacity to feel normal emotions. He has felt fearful emotions too intensely and too long.

It is a mistake for this person to search for and try to force normal feeling. He must wait for it to return, as it inevitably does. It is as if his normal emotions are frozen and he must wait for them to thaw. One woman in particular complained that for months she had felt no contact with her husband and two children. After six weeks' treatment away from the family, they were due to visit her. She immediately began to worry about whether she would feel closer to them now. I explained that she was making an issue of the situation by worrying so much about it. She had thought she had lost contact with the family for so long that the habit had become established and it was most unlikely that she would find it changed in six weeks, especially while she watched the situation so anxiously. *She must be prepared to wait for more time to pass and not record and demand progress from herself each day during their visit.* Actually, reconciled to waiting longer, she would be freed of much tension and anxiety and might therefore surprise herself by finding that they were once more all happy together.

IMAGINED STRANGENESS
IN THE BEHAVIOR OF OTHERS

Because of a feeling of withdrawal a person with nervous illness may feel so much outside the family circle that his imagination can fabricate a most emotionally involved situation from little. The woman just described, as well as thinking herself unable to contact her family, had imagined that the children no longer wanted her and would even be better off without her. Given enough time, she was likely to project herself into a variety of odd situations.

I pointed out that the children's behavior only reflected her own. They felt strange because she was acting strangely by being so conscious of, and making them conscious of, everything they said or did. If she could bring herself to be just "Mom," get their meals, talk with their friends as she used to, and cease analyzing how they felt and acted towards her, they would soon settle gratefully into being the natural children they had always been. This was what they wanted most.

Too Much Contact

In contrast with a lack of contact, some nervously ill mothers complain of being too aware of the family. They say, "It is not fair that the sick mother should be made to feel that everyone else's happiness depends on her. Why must it always be the mother's effort to make happiness for everybody? Why can't they try to make me happy for a change? As soon as I get ill they all go to pieces!"

The answer is simple. When Mother is well, she is the cord that binds the family together. When she is ill, the cord slackens, the family feels at a loose end and keeps looking to her to put things right again. They never think to change places with Mother and do a little cord pulling themselves. They just sigh miserably and wait for the hand that rocked the cradle to start rocking again. I said to one young girl, "There's plenty of food in the refrigerator, so what are you grousing about?" She answered, "I don't like just going to the fridge and getting something to eat, I like having Mom with me while I eat!" When she is well, this is Mother's life and that is how she wants it; when ill, it is still Mother's life and that is how she gets it!

Acting in a Dream

One mother was explaining to me over the telephone how difficult it was for her to accept the feeling of unreality she had toward her daughter. She said that even when she kissed her good night, it was as if she were kissing nothing, acting in a dream. She said it was like the feeling she had had coming out of an anesthetic. While we were talking I heard a great commotion beside her telephone. Suddenly the mother said "Jenny! For heaven's sake, go outside this very minute! I've had just about as much of your noise as I can stand this morning!"

When I pointed out that she had just experienced a very real moment of exasperation, she saw my point. I showed her that she had many very real moments with her daughter, but that she was so used to them they hardly registered. It was the frightening "unreal" moments that registered and blotted out the others, because she gave them all her attention.

She Didn't Kiss the Pillow

I also pointed out that when she kissed her daughter good night, she always managed to kiss her on the right place, the cheek. She didn't kiss the pillow. There was more reality in this unreal moment than she supposed. She saw the point there also. However, she will probably need much more reassurance than this until she is finally cured. In her anxious state, her emotional reaction to thought is so strong that it soon replaces the peace my explanation brings. I understand and expect this. So does she, so half our battle is won.

The Cause Must Be Very Deep Seated for Me

When the cause of feeling unreal is explained as no more than the natural result of too much anxious brooding, a nervously ill person may be so relieved that he may lose his fear of it and the sudden release from fear may make him feel more real, more part of the outside world than he has felt before. This newly gained feeling of reality may not last long. The experience of feeling unreal is so recent, it is only natural that it will return again. Memory alone will bring it back, and when it does return, so many make the mistake of once more becoming upset by it and thinking that the cause, for them, must be very deep seated indeed. A nervously ill person is *so easily bluffed by his feelings of the moment because they are so hard to bear and therefore seem so important.*

Strange Feelings in Nervous Illness Have No Real Significance

Very strange feelings may momentarily, from time to time, sweep over the nervously ill, and recovery lies in *passing right through these moments,* again and again if necessary, until they no longer matter. Strange feelings in nervous illness have no real significance, although they can be very disturbing. Recovery does not lie in trying to switch them off, tranquilize them away, or avoid them. Recovery lies in going right through them with utter acceptance in as relaxed a way as possible.

"That's My Problem, Doctor. I Can't Relax."

When I describe this procedure to some people, they immediately answer, "Now that's my problem, Doctor. I can't relax. I couldn't possibly do what you ask." My answer is always the same: "If you cannot relax your body at this stage (and I do understand this), you can at least relax your attitude to your illness."

So, if a feeling of unreality is part of your illness, be prepared to work with it, live with it, without being too impressed by it. It is not in the least important, is even usual in the circumstances. So, feel as unreal as your present state demands. Acceptance calms, tension is relaxed, and interest in the outside world gradually returns. At least you become more outward, than inward, bound.

Talking About You

It is easy for a person with nervous illness, because of a feeling of withdrawal, to become sensitive and suspicious. He may think his friends are talking about him, and they sometimes are. They notice his strained, unkempt appearance, his absent-mindedness, and they worry, so that when he re-enters a room he has just left, it is quite likely that sometimes the conversation will cease abruptly.

Do not be disconcerted by, or question, what you think is strangeness in the behavior of others toward you. Accept it all. Shrug your shoulders and think, "I am not going to be silly. It will all come right in time. Time will fix it." It will.

Look ahead to the peace of recovery and let time carry you there.

So:

When you walk through the streets wondering if you will ever be in the same world as the passers-by, remember that you will be there just as soon as you lose interest in your world of fear.

Do not try to force normal feeling; let time bring it back to you.

If others seem to act strangely toward you, practice shrugging your shoulders.

17

Obsession

Obsession experienced during nervous illness is characterized by repeated, compulsive thoughts or actions. The victim may suffer from more than one obsession and may, indeed, be in such a receptive state from fatigue that almost any repelling thought may cling and become obsessive.

"IF ONLY I COULD FORGET THE WRETCHED THING!"

If obsession is part of your illness, perhaps you are endeavoring to cure yourself by trying to forget it, and you have found that the more you try to do so the more firmly it clings. You think, "If only I could forget the wretched thing!" and rush around agitatedly trying to force forgetfulness.

You will never lose your obsession while you are trying so hard to do so. In fact, you yourself have established it by trying to push it out of your mind—in other words, by fighting it. When you fight this way, *you emphasize the obsession and keep it more vividly in your consciousness*. Fear has made it such an important part of your daily life, how could it disappear quickly?

To illustrate how difficult it is to forget on order, I ask a patient to close his eyes and imagine he sees a plate of green apples. After a minute or two, when he should have the apples well in mind, I ask him to keep his eyes closed and think of something else. When I ask later of what he thought, he usually answers, "A plate of green apples." Of course there is always the person who says otherwise, but the majority admit they continued to see a plate of green apples.

This "Thing" Will Not Seem So Terrible

The more we concentrate on forgetting, the less likely we are to forget. So, if you have obsessions, do not try to force forgetfulness. *You must accept them and be prepared to live with them for the time being.* When you decide to do this, you will feel a certain peace and this "thing" will not seem so terrible. Acceptance banishes the nightmarish quality of obsession so that you gradually lose fear of it, and with fear gone, interest goes and you either forget or remembrance holds no terror. *This is the surest and most permanent way to cure obsessions.*

It is also possible to be freed from obsession by removing yourself from the source of its origin. For example, a woman who had an obsession about crossing the main street of her town had occasion to leave the state for six months. When she returned she was delighted to find the obsession gone. Now, although she had lost it, she did not understand how, and was thus vulnerable to future obsessions and especially to the return of this one. I want to teach you how to understand and cure yourself without running away, so that you will be invulnerable to obsession forever.

"What if I Hurt My Child?"

It helps to understand obsession if you can trace its cause. The nurse tortured by the urge to throw the baby in her arms out of the window at the hospital had originally been standing beside a window, holding a baby, and had thought, as could any one of us, "Wouldn't it be terrible if I threw this child out!" In her state of mental and emotional fatigue this thought made such a searing impression that it stayed with her to become an obsession, which nearly distracted her.

She said she found it more and more difficult not to shudder and clutch the baby tightly each time she passed a window, and that the harder she fought against this impulse the stronger it seemed to become.

I explained to her that trying consciously to push this thought from her mind was the surest way to embed it more firmly there, and that she had no real wish to harm the child; indeed this was the last thing she would ever do. Her real wish was simply to be rid of the obsessive idea. She had made much of nothing by continuing to fight, and be afraid of, what had been no more than a very ordinary fleeting thought. She said, "You mean that while I was so tired the idea stuck in my mind, and because I became frightened of it, it stuck even harder?" She had described the situation exactly.

EVERY TIME SHE PASSED A WINDOW

I helped her to understand that to lose her obsession she must be prepared for a while to be reminded of it every time she passed by a window in the hospital. How could it be otherwise? She had suffered so much beside those windows, how could the memory fade quickly? But I stressed that *if she were prepared to accept these thoughts, put up with them temporarily, and not fight them, they would become unimportant and then, when that happened, they would gradually leave her.*

To see an obsession as no more than habit born from fear and fatigue robs it of its fear-inspiring quality, and with fear gone only memory remains. Time is all that is needed to fade memory.

THE PERSON WITH A
COMPULSION TO WASH HIS HANDS

A person with a compulsion to wash his hands could do so for hours without much fatigue *if he did so willingly*. It is the despair, the tension, the fear that accompany the obsession that tire to a point where reasoning becomes difficult and thought becomes compulsive. *If obeyed without fear, even such a tormenting obsession as this would gradually subside and eventually disappear, be cured.*

THOUGHTS BOUND WITHIN HIMSELF

Each obsession just described was peculiar to a particular person. However, there is an obsession caused by constant introspection that is shared by many sufferers from nervous illness. Introspection may produce intense mental fatigue, which brings to the sufferer a feeling of having his thought so bound within himself that even when he tries to be interested in other things he may find that he cannot free his thoughts sufficiently from himself to do so. He may try to work, read, or talk, only to find his thoughts reverting inward every few moments. This may give him such a feeling of enclosure within himself that he becomes conscious of his own actions, as if he cannot divorce his mind from them. He thinks that he will go crazy unless he can put an end to this misery.

He may spend months suffering these frequent, intermittent recessions of thought, perhaps trying to carry on responsible work at the same time, but feeling caught in a trap from which he cannot escape. There may be days when the habit leaves him, only to return and throw him into deeper despair.

GAZING AT THE CEILING

When alone the sufferer is not so aware of his obsession (we can call it an obsession) because there are fewer outside interests to divert his attention from himself. It is when he must meet people that his misery begins. So he may avoid company and stay in his room. Even reading is no help because, as he reads, his thoughts turn inward, until he hardly knows what he is reading and feels like throwing the book away. Small wonder if, when his mother peeps anxiously into his room, she finds him with his head buried in the pillow or gazing stolidly at the ceiling.

LET YOUR THOUGHTS PLAY TRICKS

First, understand that this obsession is no more than a manifestation of intense mental fatigue. Therefore sleep as much as you can. If not very successful at this, do not immediately panic and think that you now have no chance of recovery. *Following the second instruction alone will cure you.*

Second, let your thoughts play their tricks as they will. Concentrating hard on trying to forget oneself is merely another way of concentrating anxiously on oneself. *Do not try to forget yourself.* Do not try to force your way back into anything. Accept yourself as you are now, with all your strange thoughts. It does not matter what you think about, or *how much you dwell on yourself, providing you do not do it anxiously.* That is the key. It is the anxiety that tenses, sensitizes, *not the thoughts.* Accept your thoughts, whatever they are, as part of your ordinary thinking. Do not make the mistake of believing that there are certain thoughts you must not think, dare not think, as if there are parts of your brain you must not use. Use them all, even those that may hold an obsession; *but use them willingly, shrink from none of them.* None of us ever completely forgets himself. You are only much more conscious of yourself than you normally would be. This is not important, although it can be devastatingly frustrating.

Accept your habit of introspection with as little frustration as possible. You may be often disappointed in the beginning. Be prepared for this. Thoughts may be fantastic when you are anxious. You may go chasing them to see how odd they can become, and the stranger, more unreal they seem, the more you may push on, as if compelled to find out the worst, compelled to challenge the worst. And do not make the mistake of thinking that this is mental. You are merely once more afraid of fear, but this time in one of its most bewildering and upsetting guises.

Thoughts Turn Inward More Lightly

Understanding your condition as brainfag that will gradually disappear with enough sleep, acceptance, and occupation; realizing that you are not going mad and that many before you have felt this way, will release you from some fear and tension, so that your thoughts will turn inward more lightly, will be less clinging, until they are no more than a touch, and the smallest interest will be enough to make you forget the habit.

However, this habit, although accepted with resignation, may continue to come for a while and, as it can be most exhausting, do not hesitate occasionally to seek the solace of solitude. In this way you will find some respite. Also, do not force yourself to read while reading is a strain. The time will soon come when you will be able to read without effort.

The question could be asked, "If he is not to read now, how can he read this book of yours, Doctor?" Anything about nerves is so compellingly interesting to a sufferer from nervous illness that it holds his attention, and inward thinking, if it does not completely cease, at least fades into insignificance.

A German woman with this type of obsession described it graphically and told how a friend helped to cure her. When she felt one of these exasperating periods approaching, she would run to her friend and say, "It's coming again, Maria. It's starting again!" and Maria would answer, "Let it come, Anna. Don't try to fight it. Go with it and it will pass." Wise Maria.

Tape Recordings

To help my patients with obsession I make tape recordings of their interviews with me and they then use these whenever they need reassurance and guidance, which is often: much oftener than the weekly or fortnightly visit usually allowed. Indeed, help may be needed hourly in the beginning by a person trying to cure himself of obsessive habit.

So, to cure your obsession:

> Accept and do not try to force forgetfulness.
> Stop fighting.
> Let time pass while you do this.

Once more, the familiar pattern of recovery.

18

Depression

DEPRESSION IN THE COURSE OF NERVOUS ILLNESS

A person emotionally exhausted by months of worry may gradually become apathetic. Apathy may gradually turn to depression, or depression can strike suddenly in one overwhelming wave. The sudden, swift descent of depression can be a shattering experience if its victim is taken unaware. Whether depression descends gradually or suddenly, it is one of the worst phases of nervous illness because it robs so many of the wish to recover. However, most people rise above depression enough to hope for recovery. I assure such people they can recover, *however deep their depression.* For those people who have completely lost interest in recovery, electric (shock) treatment is sometimes advised. Lest a depressed person think I advise shock treatment for all depressed people, I hasten to repeat, however depressed you may be, if you wish to recover *without shock treatment,* you can. Let there be no misunderstanding about this. Modern anti-depressant drugs help, but these, like sedatives, should be prescribed only by a doctor.

WE THRASH THE SELF-STARTER

Depression is a body's expression of emotional exhaustion. I could liken our emotional reserves to the battery of a car. If we thrash the self-starter, the battery may go flat. If we thrash our emotional battery with fear, despair, it may eventually become flat and we feel apathetic, depressed. Just as a car battery will recharge itself if we drive without thrashing the self-starter or leaving the lights on unnecessarily, so will our emotional battery recharge itself if we stop thrashing our body with those expensive emotions, fear and despair.

SITTING ABOUT THE HOUSE
WATCHING THE HOURS PASS

The nervously ill person needs to understand what I have been teaching and must be prepared to accept his depression as well as his nervous symptoms, while letting time pass to bring recovery, but it is essential that he has necessary medication, encouragement, and occupation.

I have seen people on the verge of recovery deteriorate severely when suddenly deprived of occupation. They should not attempt to recover from nervous illness sitting about the house watching the days pass, trying to fill each hour as it comes. They must have an organized program so that they can look ahead and know how each day will be filled.

I sometimes find it difficult to convince a patient's family of the importance of occupation. They have no conception of how long an idle hour can seem to the nervously ill, depressed person. His tired mind, turned inward on itself, is conscious of every moment as it passes, so that an hour seems an eternity to him and tension increases until it seems unbearable. This situation is exasperating to a doctor, because he knows that idleness, tension, and depression make a formidable trio that could have been avoided if he had had the family's co-operation in finding occupation. It is absolutely essential for a nervously ill person that thoughts be claimed by outside interests, so that time passes more quickly, the strain is eased, and depression thus relieved.

SMALL, HAPPY, DAILY EXPERIENCE

Normally our spirits are kept up by small, happy, daily experiences of which we are hardly aware. For example, while we wash up and try to decide whether to make the beds next or hose the garden, we handle the smooth china we like and notice the sun shining on the scarlet geraniums on the window sill. Our heart lifts up, and when we go into the bedroom, it is with much less than our usual annoyance that we remove the sleeping cat from the bed. The nervously ill person if shown a garden full of geraniums would probably stare and say, "Geraniums? What geraniums?" His preoccupation with his problems and himself deadens his powers of observation and so bars entry to these small joys.

So many of these small, happy experiences are waiting to help lift your spirit. The future is not as black as you may think. You do not need some great happiness to bring back joy in living. The little things will do that, as soon as you have eyes to see them.

THE LONELY PEACE OF SOLITUDE

Working out of doors is particularly recommended for depression. The brightness, the expanse of sky, the absence of restraining walls, the movement, all help to keep spirits raised and troubles in proportion. The depressed person with no inner source of joy for support depends almost entirely on cheerful environment to help him. A melancholic atmosphere is almost unendurable. Indeed, his reaction to sadness is so exaggerated that a slightly depressing situation may seem tragic to him. And this reaction is quick. A nervously ill woman went to stay at the seaside. She arrived at dusk on a windy, gray day. As she stepped from the automobile a gusty wind from the beach brought the sound of the local amateur band practicing mournfully nearby and a handful of crows circled overhead calling their baleful, "Caw! Caw! Caw!" The depressing effect was instantaneous and shattering. She felt her heart sink into her boots and she said it took two days of sunshine to recover it.

It is often better for a depressed person to sit in the local movies or have a meal in a busy shop or restaurant than to rest in the lonely peace of solitude. Brightness and diversion help to hold the interest and support the flagging spirit.

RESPITE MAY HIGHLIGHT SUFFERING

Some people with nervous illness refuse to visit the movies for several reasons. They say that the feeling of unreality they experience there makes them more aware of the frightening unreal feeling of their illness. Others say that to hear so many people laughing happily only emphasizes their own isolation and misery; while others find that although they can lose themselves in a movie, to come back to the hard light of reality when the performance is over and face their condition again can be such a contrast, such a shock, that their illness seems more overwhelming and hopeless than ever. The respite only highlights their suffering.

COWED BY A THOUGHT

It is such strange experiences as these that make nervous illness a bewildering maze and keep it alive as a constant source of torture. To get out of the maze you must go forward and meet these experiences when they come. Do not try to avoid them, but do not challenge them and seek them out unnecessarily. Merely accept them and be prepared to let more time pass until you can face them without suffering. Remember, the blow that strikes as you are recalled from temporary forgetfulness of your suffering is *no more than a thought. You are being cowed by a thought.*

Do not be bluffed by a thought. Why not think a comforting thought instead of a frightening one? This may not be easy at first, but practice makes it easier. Instead of thinking "Dear God, the illness! Will I never forget? Will I never escape?" you can think "I forgot it for a moment. I won't panic because I remember it again. I'll think of it as calmly as I can, and gradually remembering will not be so painful." Actually, as you recover, forgetting and then remembering changes to a feeling of joy, joy at remembering that you are recovering. So do not be too disturbed *now* when you forget yourself for a while, and afterward remember your illness again. Accept even that. You cannot hope ever to forget your illness completely. How could you? If you saw a murder, could you ever completely forget what you saw? Never. So your ultimate aim is *to remember without too much fear*. How much of your illness is built up from no more than frightening thoughts, frightening memories?

NERVOUS EXPERIENCE AT THE MOVIES

Facing your illness after momentarily forgetting it is an experience you may have to go through many times daily. As I just explained, this will be less painful as you face it with acceptance. But I do not mean that you must face every particular detail that frightens you. It may be wiser to avoid certain experiences while sensitized, especially if facing them serves no useful purpose. For example, one woman had had an especially depressing, upsetting, nervous experience at the movies and she said that she now had only to see the outside of a theater to have devastating reactions. She had made herself worse by going especially to the movies "to try to conquer" this feeling.

I explained that her reactions were severe now only because of present oversensitization of her adrenalin-releasing nerves and that visiting the movies in the future would not always affect her this way. While it was necessary for her to face, unmask, and then float past fears that must be met, going to the movies served no useful purpose at the moment and it would be better to avoid such unnecessary suffering until her reactions calmed down. But I emphasized that she must avoid *sensibly, hopefully, not fearfully,* knowing that eventually she would have only a memory of her earlier disturbance. She must realize that avoidance now was merely to save reopening *a healing wound.* She would not recover so quickly if she fearfully avoided the movies, or if she went there tensely prepared to "fight this thing." Can you appreciate the difference between these two approaches? It is one of the keys to recovery.

LIVING ALONE

When they are well, people live alone successfully because they have the energy and interest to take part in the life about them. When nervously ill, living alone may seem unbearably tragic and depressing. I strongly advise you not to live alone while ill. By all means leave home temporarily and stay with friends or even go to a boardinghouse: anywhere where you can live with people. But do not make any arrangements now to relinquish your home permanently. You will feel differently about it when you are recovered, and homes are not easy to find. Make no impulsive, irretrievable step.

DEPRESSION IS YOU, NOT THE WORLD

Also, a depressed person should remember that depression is a physical feeling expressing the extreme tiredness of his emotions. As you stop flogging yourself with fear, fight, and flight from fear, you become less tired and depression gradually lifts.

Above all, remember that depression is you, and it is not the world that is so terrible. Depression is an illness, just as influenza is an illness, and nature is waiting as readily to cure one as the other if you will let her. But depression works in such a vicious circle; the memory of yesterday's suffering makes such a bad start for today. You can get outside that circle by saying, "All right, yesterday was a bad day. Today may not be good either, but as the days go by, they will gradually improve if I let them." When you can say this and mean it, you will see a miracle happen.

Remember:

However deep your depression, you can recover.

Depression is a temporary illness.

Modern anti-depressant drugs are helpful.

Keep off that bed in the daytime and be occupied in the company of others.

Have a planned program of occupation.

When respite highlights suffering, review your thoughts and substitute hope for despair.

Once more, depression is an illness; nature is waiting to cure you.

DEPRESSION UNACCOMPANIED BY OTHER NERVOUS ILLNESS

Many people suffer with a habit of recurring depression, and yet they cannot be said to be nervously ill in the same way as the person just described. These people respond so quickly, so acutely to a mildly depressing atmosphere that they have but to see lowering clouds at dusk or hear rooks in the belfry to feel their spirits literally sink. Usually their attention is soon distracted and they quickly recover. However, they need have only a few such experiences in close succession to be convinced that a bout of depression is on its way. They immediately become apprehensive, afraid. Who wouldn't? There is nothing quite so depressing as depression. And because reaction usually comes when they are overtired, the added strain of apprehension and fear drains their emotions still further and so makes depression more likely to descend.

Let us look closely at such a person and see the mistakes made, mistakes that not only invite depression but prolong its visit. You will see that these mistakes arise very much from first trying to fight the thought of approaching depression and then fighting depression itself.

I Choose a Woman Rather Than a Man

Let us look at a housewife who suffers from depression. I choose a woman rather than a man, because a woman's life at home is more conducive to depression than a man's life in the outside world. I also choose a woman who has frequent bouts of rather severe depression, so that the lurking shadow of depression may never be far away. Of course what I say applies also to men, especially men whose work demands emotional energy, for example, men in advertising, artists, writers, musicians.

The Fight Has Begun

First, this housewife, whom we will now consider, dreads and fears depression, so that when she feels one of her bouts approaching she may rush feverishly through her work, trying to fill each moment so that she will have little time to think about that hovering cloud. *The fight has begun.* When she finishes her work, she is so afraid to be alone with her thoughts, her feelings, she's off visiting one friend after another. She's off to the supermarket, away to a movie, rushing here, rushing there, trying to forget the state she is in, trying to push away that threatening cloud.

"Is It Still There?"

But all the time, even when out, she watches herself apprehensively, thinking, "Is it still there? I hope it won't come back when I get home!" It is difficult to forget something while trying so hard to forget. The best way to remember is to try too hard to forget. So, by feverishly rushing, trying to ward off depression, this woman may succeed only in emphasizing its threat.

PUTTING ON AN ACT BEFORE THE FAMILY

Also, agitated rushing is tiring, so she becomes over-tired, tense, and irritable. Putting on an act before the family is also a strain. So the tension mounts and gradually brings sensitization, so that the wave of fear she feels when she thinks of approaching depression becomes more and more acute. She feels this spasm in the pit of her stomach, in the exact spot where she feels the sinking sensation of depression. There is so little to choose between these two feelings, fear and depression, that as the fear mounts, she translates this feeling of fear into the feeling of depression itself and is finally convinced that depression has arrived.

THE BARRAGE FROM FAMILY AND FRIENDS

At this point she despairs, and despair is the finishing touch. She has but to feel one flash of utter despair to admit at last to herself and to the family that she really is having one of her bouts. Now comes the barrage from family and friends, "Pull yourself together, Mother. Snap out of it. Fight it, Mother!" As if she hasn't been fighting it for days, weeks and getting nowhere except more deeply enmeshed. However, she starts once more on the old routine, rushing here, rushing there, fighting this, fighting that, trying to snap out of it, trying to rise above it. She takes anti-depressant pills each morning to pick herself up, sedatives each afternoon to calm herself down—a pill for this and a pill for that.

While out visiting, she may sometimes feel almost happy and for a moment may forget her depression; but when she thinks of it again, the contrast, between the cheerfulness she has been feeling while happily distracted and the sinking feeling that comes as she remembers the state she is really in, is so striking that her spirits sink immediately, even deeper than before. The fight seems hopeless. What is the use of forgetting when remembering is such pain? So she may return home more depressed, more discouraged than when she set out.

Sometimes she may start for home feeling fine, only to find that the very sight of the house throws her into deep despair. While she is so easily cast down, it is difficult to remember that, in the past, depression always lifted. With each new bout, there is always the fear that this one will stay.

ONE MORNING, LESS FOREBODING, MORE INTEREST

Depression always passes because, as I have already explained, it is a state of emotional depletion, and as emotional reserves rebuild, spirits automatically rise. Emotional reserves do replenish themselves, even during depression. So one morning, despite herself, this woman will waken to find less foreboding, more interest. From past experience she knows this sign well. It means that this bout of depression is on its way out at last. She immediately takes heart, fears it less, becomes less tense, is even prepared to wait patiently for it to go completely.

AIDS IN ABOLISHING DEPRESSION

Now this is a story of complete mismanagement, mismanagement that not only establishes recurring bouts of depression as a habit, but also prolongs each bout.

What should a person do to prevent depression coming or, if it has already descended, to help lift himself out of it? Change, interesting occupation, company are well-known aids in abolishing depression. They divert attention from those expensive emotions, fear and despair, and so give opportunity for natural healing. But change, interesting occupation, and company are not always available. Most people, especially housewives, must recover in their usual routine. So what can they do to help themselves? Indeed, if you suffer from recurring depression what can you do to help yourself?

THOSE DEVITALIZING
EMOTIONS, FEAR AND DESPAIR

When you first feel that sinking feeling of depression, you should have the courage *to relax toward it* and let it come. Don't tense yourself against it in fear, in dread. If you feel apathetic, depressed, try to understand that this is a reaction that has been fostered by habit and memory and encouraged by emotional and mental fatigue. Don't run tensely, blindly from the thought of depression with your mind closed against it in fear. Don't drain your emotions still further by indulging in those devitalizing emotions, fear and despair, especially despair. Work at a steady pace, your usual pace, so that you can take time to think calmly of yourself; think calmly of your work, and especially take time to think calmly about depression. I do not mean that you should sit and wallow in depression. By all means take every opportunity that offers to help cheer yourself; help recharge your emotional batteries, but *do this at a normal pace, at a steady pace.*

ACCEPTANCE WILL CUSHION
THE SHOCK OF REMEMBERING

If while out you forget your depression for a while, don't be too cast down when you remember it again. If you accept that your batteries are flat for the moment and that emotions will swing up one moment and down the next, your acceptance will cushion the shock of remembering depression, and this will protect your emotions from your own onslaught upon them and give your body a chance to heal itself, to replenish its emotional stores.

It takes courage to relax toward depression, one might say to rest in depression, and not try to fight it by seeking salvation in hectic, tiring distraction. To face, accept, and quietly work on *at a normal pace*—that is the secret, and it will work a miracle if done without fear.

19

That Dreaded Morning Feeling

Waking in the morning deserves special attention. It is the worst time of day to most people with nervous illness, not only because it brings another day to face, but because it may also so disappointingly fail to fulfill the expectations of the previous night. There are days when the sufferer feels comparatively well and by evening has convinced himself that he really is getting better at last. He goes to bed cheerful and optimistic only to find, on waking the next morning, that the previous day's improvement seems but a dream.

THE SAME OLD HEART OF LEAD

It is strange how the morning has the disconcerting habit of apparently paying little regard to the improvement of the day before. People are disappointed and bewildered when, after going to bed fairly cheerful, they wake the next morning to find the same old heart of lead, the same depression, the same churning stomach, the same difficulty in facing the day, the same desire to switch off their engine and pull the blankets over their head. It is as if the morning lags behind the pace of their recovery.

It is not easy to find a satisfactory explanation for this dreaded morning feeling. It may be that consciousness steals upon you before you have time to marshal your defenses. If you have had oblivion in sleep, the

moment of waking—bringing the return of cold reality
—may strike like a blow across the face and your spirits may sink before you have time to save them. Or it
may be that sleep relaxes an overtired body to a point
beyond normal relaxation, and this is as hard to bear
as tension. Whatever it is, I do know that when you
wake in the morning feeling that the world is not such
a bad place you are well on the way to recovery.

The suffering felt on waking must be understood,
almost expected, but not magnified. Don't let it bluff
you. *A difficult morning need not mean a difficult
day.*

Rise When You Wake

To cope with this morning feeling, *you must rise as
soon as you wake.* The longer you lie steeped in misery the harder it will be to pull yourself out of it. I
fully understand how difficult early rising can be, but
it can be done, even though it may mean literally
dragging your body out of bed. "I leap out of bed,"
said one woman. But very few people with nervous
illness are prepared to leap out of bed. It is enough if,
as soon as you open your eyes, you rise, however slowly, have a shower, and then go and make a cup of tea.
You will find that cheerful music helps to lift you out
of the early-morning doldrums, so have a radio beside your bed. The family may not appreciate an early-
morning concert, but when they know it is part of
your treatment they usually co-operate.

After music, shower, and tea, you can lie more peacefully in bed until the family stirs. You may prefer to go
for a walk rather than return to bed. So much the better. The main thing is *to make some quick efforts as
soon as you open your eyes, so that the early-morning depression cannot establish itself.* Having done
this, you will not so easily slip back into depression
again. At least it will not seem so overwhelming as it
might have done had you stayed in bed with the blankets over your head. Be prepared to greet the mornings
this way until waking becomes easier and you know

you can lie in peace without the aid of music, shower, or tea.

"THE BODILY FUNCTIONS AREN'T WORKING YET!"

When I advised one young woman to rise as soon as she woke, she remonstrated, "But the bodily functions aren't working! How could I get out of bed before the bodily functions work? It sometimes takes hours for mine to get going!" I assured her that her "bodily functions" would work more quickly in response to command than to coaxing, especially when their owner lay in bed engrossed in the coaxing. Admittedly the first half hour may feel deadly, and it is from this that most people shrink. However, after a while the way becomes easier, helped by the prompt rising.

So don't listen to any excuse you may make yourself to lie a little longer. *Leave that bed as soon as you wake.*

HAVE COMPANY

Having someone congenial to talk to on waking is a great comfort, and do not think yourself a coward if you would like some member of the family sleeping in the room with you. This is good treatment and I sometimes advise it. To see another person on waking brings a feeling of reassurance and reality, and a few spoken words can be as balm to a troubled mind.

At least place your bed so that you can see out of the window when you wake and are not forced to look at the same spot on the ceiling, or at the same old dressing gown hanging up behind the door. To see something moving outside, if only the boughs of a tree, is a distraction and somehow helps you to feel more normal.

EARLY-MORNING SEDATIVE

If you wake at four o'clock or thereabouts, it becomes a problem to decide whether to take another sleeping pill, get up, or just lie and "stew." Even though the family may be willing to suffer the disturbance, four o'clock is too early for you to begin the day. You are left with too many hours to fill in until the household stirs. So I advise patients to take a little more sedative. For this purpose, a tablet is prescribed that acts quickly and yet does not leave much hangover. Even if you do not sleep again, the tablet is calming and you can more easily lie and wait until it is time to rise. When I advise rising as soon as you wake, I do not mean to do so while the moon is still shining and the owl still sitting on the fence.

A Change of View

You may be surprised how helpful it is to change your bedroom or even the position of your bed or the curtains in your room. To wake each morning and see the same curtains with the same pattern, of which you know every detail, reminds you so vividly of all the other mornings of suffering, that you may seem to be dragged back into the quagmire before you can save yourself. Change refreshes—even such small changes as these. As mentioned, change acts like a mild shock that temporarily arrests your attention and draws it away from yourself and so helps you to feel more normal. Even a short respite from suffering is heartening.

So, should you wake with that dreaded morning feeling:

Rise immediately, have a shower, make a hot drink, find some cheerful music on the radio, or, if time permits, go for a walk.

Do not be too impressed by the necessity to lie in bed until your "bodily functions get going"; rise and get them going yourself.

Place your bed so that you can see outside on waking.

Change your bedroom if possible; at least occasionally move the furniture in your room to make a change.

Above all, accept and do not be discouraged by the mornings while waiting for them to improve, remembering that a difficult morning need not mean a difficult day.

20

Sleeplessness

By nightfall some sufferers from nervous illness feel so much better and brighter than in the morning that they almost convince themselves they are cured. Others, particularly those with problems, dread the night. They lie in a bed of panic and sweat, with terrifying thoughts racing through their minds, waiting for sedation to calm them. They are afraid to be in the room alone and dread switching off the light.

If you are in this state, sedation is indeed a boon, but there are other ways to woo sleep.

First, understand that your fears are terrifying *only because your body is in a sensitized state,* shooting off exaggerated responses, where normally you would feel perhaps no more than a vague disturbance. *Your problems are not as terrible as your tired, sensitized body would have you believe.* If you were not having such upsetting reactions at the thought of them you could probably cope with them. Therefore, try to see your panic for what it is, *the exaggerated response of sensitized nerves* and not necessarily an expression of the magnitude of your problem. Make yourself as comfortable in bed as you can, relax to the best of your ability, then examine the feeling of panic and be *prepared to let it sweep over you. Relax and go with it.* Do not shrink from it or try to control it.

You will find that if you can do this, the waves of panic will settle into being a hot, sore feeling in the pit of your stomach. You can get so used to this feeling that you can drop off to sleep with it there.

Your own thoughts may bring this panic, or it may sweep over you without apparent cause. If your thoughts are to blame, recognize that they are only thoughts; although, coming as they do so charged with fear, they may appear as monsters. Recognize that they are only thoughts and let them float away. *Release them. Let them go. Do not clutch them.*

When you decide to face panic and see it through, you feel some relief, and this brings its own relaxation and a certain amount of peace. I say a certain amount, because at first you may not be aware of a great change in the way you feel. Although there is acceptance in your mind, your body may not respond to this for a while. However, it is possible that you may be surprised at the relief you feel. This may be so great that you may find your attention wandering from yourself.

It is easy for me to say relax and accept. I know that it may be very difficult for a tense, panic-stricken person to relax, but it can be done. Remember, the panic is there only because your nerves are sensitized to it. *One spasm of fear is making you more fearful of the next,* so that each spasm seems more intense than the last. If you relax, analyze the spasms (as advised in a previous chapter), and resign yourself to having them temporarily, without adding *second* fear, you will develop an inner peace that will break the cycle of spasm-panic-spasm.

Your Mind May Feel As Weak As Water

If unsolved problems aggravate your sleeplessness, you must act and do something about solving them or coming to some compromise. I have already suggested how to do this. Sleeplessness will not pass until you have a plan that will cope at least with your major problem. Indecision and conflict leave you a prey to fear and fatigue. Your mind may literally feel as weak as water. In trying to decide, it may turn first one way and then another, until you feel incapable of mak-

ing any decision and lie floundering, sweating, and uncertain. It is this uncertainty that makes you so vulnerable to panic and sleeplessness. Hence the necessity
of having a point of view, found for you if need be, to
which your mind can cling and so rest itself and find
sleep.

How to Relax

Many articles have been written on relaxation.
Therefore I will only briefly describe here a simple
method, the nucleus of most other methods.

Lie comfortably in bed, first making sure that the
bedclothes are not too heavy. Then, beginning with
your feet and passing up to your legs, abdomen, chest,
neck, head, arms, and hands in that order, imagine
that each in turn is so heavy it feels as though it is
sinking through the mattress. Be sure to include your
jaws and tongue in this lead-laden picture.

When you first relax your abdomen you may be
more acutely conscious of its pulsation than when you
were tensely controlling it. Understand that this pulsation is no more than the action of the main artery in
your body, the aorta, in its effort to pump blood into
your legs. If you press your hand into your abdomen
you can feel this artery pulsating. Pulsating blood is
your lifeline. Why be upset by this normal, necessary
phenomenon simply because, as a result of tension, it
is more forceful than usual and you are therefore more
conscious of it?

The throbbing noise in your ear is also caused by
blood coursing through one of the larger arteries in
your head. When you hear this, instead of arranging
your pillows to try and deaden it, say to yourself,
"There goes my lifeline. Good for it! Why worry if
it's a bit loud tonight?" Relax and let it throb, and
the pumping will calm down.

Head Noises

Some people complain of a noise in their heads
like a pistol shot, which comes just as they are going

off to sleep. Be pleased if you hear this. It is a sign that your tensed muscles are relaxing and that sleep is not far away.

Others say their head seems to swing on the pillow like a pendulum. This is yet another sign that sleep is coming. Rest your head on the pillow and let the pendulum swing. It is possible to fall to sleep with it swinging, and the pendulum does you no harm. It is but a temporary upset in your balancing mechanism caused by fatigue.

LISTEN

There is yet another way to find sleep. Sometimes a tired brain can be exasperatingly overactive. You can help to calm this excessive activity by using the receptive area of your brain, that is, *by listening.* Lie and listen to outside noises. Thoughts will come while you do this, but they will not be as penetrating as when you are actively thinking, nor will they be such organized emotion-bearing thoughts. I do this after a day of pressure when it is a temptation to lie awake and relive the day's happenings or plan the next day's activities. I simply lie and listen and have trained myself to do so for longer and longer periods without thinking. Sleep eventually comes. The well-known suggestion of counting sheep is an example of this principle. When watching imaginary sheep we use the visual receptive area of our brain and spare the thinking area. In practice, listening to outside sounds is much more effective than watching sheep, which few seem to find satisfactory.

Of course, I know there are people whose nerves are so agitated, and for whom stress is such torture, that sleep so induced would be too slow in coming. These people, if not given sleep quickly, face the next day more exhausted than when they lay down the previous night. They need a strong, quickly acting sedative and should consult their doctor about it.

But I emphasize that sedation alone will not cure. The patient must be prepared to *accept and float,* must have settled his problems or have found a compromise and must now be using sedatives mainly to overcome the residual tension in his body brought on by weeks, even years, of previous suffering and fighting.

THE JIGSAW PUZZLE

The nervously ill person has the habit of frustrating sleep by lying in bed at night trying to "work things out." He endeavors to unravel why such and such occurred today and to decide what he could have done to avoid it. I remember a woman who came to me late one night to tell me she "had the answer." She said, eyes bright with excitement, "I know why my arms ache and keep me awake. I shouldn't have typed so much today. I overdid it." She had spent hours working that one out.

Don't lie in bed trying to fit the pieces of your illness together like reconstructing a jigsaw puzzle. You excite and disturb yourself unnecessarily, because you will make a different picture each night. You don't have to trace your way out of nervous illness step by step. Practice masterly inactivity, and when you lay your head on the pillow at night try to accept everything and float off to sleep. If you do this, sleep will come in spite of your having typed too much during the day!

CHILDREN

A nervously sick mother with small children finds it difficult to get enough sleep. The children so often wake and demand attention just as she is drifting off. Noises heard as a tense person is on the verge of sleep can cause an electrifying reaction, disturbing, almost painful, and capable of bringing the sleeper back to full consciousness in a matter of seconds.

I explain to husbands the benefit of uninterrupted sleep for a sick wife and that no woman with severe nervous illness should have the responsibility of looking after children, especially at night. Unfortunately some men are difficult to convince. While the wife can drag herself around, he expects her to. This is understandable, for she may look well enough and may have little more than a frayed temper to show for her illness. As for finding help for his wife, who wants to look after another woman's children unless well paid, and where is he to get the money to do this? Goodness knows he has spent enough on his wife already!

Social service agencies may provide help in some circumstances. However, I usually advise the sick mother to leave home for two months (not one), if possible, and not to think she is "deserting the ship" by so doing.

If it is impossible for a mother to leave home or obtain help, she has no alternative but to accept her lot with as little frustration as possible, remembering that it is not so much rising and attending to the children that continues to keep her awake as lying in bed afterward, burning up with the thought of how she would like to hang, draw, and quarter every one of them, starting with the peaceful snorer at her side.

As well as philosophical acceptance, such a housewife has her relatives, good neighbors, and sedative to help her, and I have seen these work wonders. She now also has this book.

OTHER STRANGE HURDLES

Going to sleep may be beset by other strange hurdles. If the sufferer has had a series of sleepless nights and feels another would be more than he could bear, the very intensity of his desire for sleep is enough to make him more tense and anxious, and this becomes so upsetting that sleep is even less likely to come.

The principles of treatment stressed here meet this and each of the emergencies described above. Relax to the best of your ability, and accept the strangeness, the previous loss of sleep, the palpitations, the tension, the sweating, the panic, remembering that behind all this *nature is waiting to put you to sleep. Sleep is lurking in the background, even behind such tension.* Also remember that if sleep does not come tonight it will come tomorrow or the night after. *It will eventually come.* It has been coming nightly to mankind for thousands of years. *This habit is stronger than your power to prevent it.*

By this I do not mean that you should lie awake for hours, waiting for sleep to come. It is wiser to take a prescribed sedative and cut short the hours of tension. The frame of mind described above can be cultivated while waiting for the sedative to take effect or when you have improved and are beginning to sleep without sedation. Remember, your sedation must be prescribed and supervised by a doctor.

So, to encourage sleep:

Understand that your fears are terrifying because your body is in a sensitized state.

Relax, and let panic sweep over you; go with it, do not shrink from it.

Recognize that much of your panic is inspired by thoughts, and do not be bluffed by thoughts.

Settle your problems as soon as you can, seeking advice, if necessary.

Remember that head noises are harmless.

If your mind is overactive, lie and listen to outside sounds.

Do not excite yourself at night trying to unravel your illness; practice masterly inactivity, relax, and accept.

If you have done too much during the day, don't waste energy lying in bed worrying about it.

Remember that the habit of sleeping is stronger than your power to prevent it.

Do not hesitate to use sedatives, but remember that they must be prescribed by a doctor.

21

Difficulty in Returning Home

It is sometimes advisable to remove the patient to new surroundings to help speed recovery. However, the time eventually comes when recovery is sufficiently advanced to warrant returning home. Telling a nervously ill housewife that she is so much better she may soon return home is not always the happy task for a doctor one might suppose. I am very cautious when I mention going home to a nervously ill woman. I have seen so many make good progress away from home and then suddenly wilt when told they may soon go home.

THE FAMILY THINK
THEY HAVE DONE THEIR PART

The patient senses how critical those first few weeks back at home may be; that this is the time when she may either go forward to complete recovery, or relapse once more into illness and despair, and into a despair she senses may be more desperate than ever, because of the tantalizing glimpse of recovery she has had while away. She knows the hazards ahead only too well. She knows she is returning to the same routine that helped to keep her ill. She also knows that the family think they have done their part by doing without her; that she has had rest and treatment while away; and that they, as well as she, should now be able to forget the whole upsetting experience as soon as possible.

HER VENEER OF RECOVERY IS THIN

She understands this attitude but she fears it, because she realizes that her veneer of recovery is thin. She's had the experience of feeling on top of the world one day and imagining herself completely out of the wood, only to feel, the next day, the same old apprehension, the same distressing symptoms as strongly as ever. Experiences like these warn her that recovery will take time, and yet she knows that necessity, particularly her family's necessity, may not allow her this time. One of my patients was greeted almost at the front door with, "Thank heavens, you're home. Now we can have some decent food at last. How about a cherry pie?"

Oh yes, the housewife knows all the hazards of homecoming. Friends or relatives may put themselves out once to mind the children while she goes away, but twice? Small wonder that as the time for returning home draws near, her growing apprehension may bring relapse. Unfortunately this is sometimes interpreted by those treating her as a subconscious wish to escape into illness to avoid her responsibilities. This is so far from the truth that she becomes even more upset, because in her heart she wants nothing more than to be her old self again and get on with the job.

"MUMMY! MUMMY!"

The woman recovering away from home knows that much of her improvement came from the comfort of having her day filled with change and occupation in the company of others and, what is more, occupation *within the limits of her capacity*. Most of us, if we have a day alone at home, enjoy those moments of dawdling over a cup of tea and a magazine, enjoy just doing nothing. However, as I have so often emphasized before, doing nothing can be one of the most difficult tasks for a nervously ill person, and occupation, when it comes to the housewife, may take no heed of the limits of her capacity: for example, the overwhelming early-morning rush, the evening avalanche. One minute she is agitatedly rushing, trying to answer demands for "Mummy! Mummy!" and the next she may be wandering from room to room, staring in lonely desperation at the empty hours ahead.

"Will I Slip Back?"

Perhaps you are about to leave the hospital and the thought of going home disturbs you. You think, "How will I react to being home? Will I slip back?" If you are returning after recovering by floating and accepting, you will have an excellent idea of how to act, because the same principle applies. There must be no fighting; no spotlight turned onto your feelings; no questioning yourself, "Do I like this? Do I like that?"

It is not important how you feel when you first go home. Your feelings are bound to be mixed. You will be glad to be home; frightened to be home; scared of seeing again the places where you suffered; glad to be among the people you love and yet afraid lest you disappoint them and become ill again. *Realize that none of these feelings is permanent, and that none is therefore really important.* Admit them to yourself, but do not make much of them. Accept that you will probably have a strange mixture of feelings for a while. Who wouldn't? Talk about them with a sympathetic member of the family. Putting your fears into words will help to dispel them more quickly. But deep down, take with you the knowledge that *reconciled acceptance of all strange feelings will gradually abolish them.* You have already experienced how acceptance has calmed the sensations of illness. It will also calm these feelings of apprehension.

"Why Can't I Be Happy in My Home?"

Despite your resolutions, you may seem to deteriorate on first returning home. You may be left alone all day, and after being constantly with people while away, the contrast with the loneliness at home may at first seem too great. Also, in spite of preparing yourself for distressing memories around the house, actual contact with them can be surprisingly upsetting, and you may fail to differentiate between reality and memory; so that, as you wander from room to room, assailed by painful recollection, you may panic and think you are "slipping back." You think, "Why can't I be happy in my home? Why must it do this to me? I'm no better than I was. And yet I felt so much better while I was away. What's wrong with me?"

"As Soon As I Put My Foot upon the Stairs!"

This is the home you love, but it is also the place where you suffered deeply, and it would not be humanly possible to forget such suffering easily. You may remember the woman who said she couldn't get a "holt" on herself? Eventually she was cured and after a holiday telephoned joyously to say how well she felt and that she was coming to see me the next day. She arrived looking well enough, but did not seem as radiant as she had sounded the day before. In fact, she wore the shadow of the old frightened look, and I said, "You're surprised to find that as soon as you sat in that familiar chair, your old fears came back?" She answered, "They were back before that, Doctor! As soon as I put my foot on the stairs, they were back! What's wrong with me?"

I said, "You would be a magician if you could immediately banish the memory of suffering associated with climbing those stairs. But understand that *it is only memory* and don't be bluffed by it. Float past it, and the next time you come you will be surprised how easy it will be." She left relieved and happy.

So, if faced with a similar situation, accept that you may be at first disturbed by painful memories on returning home; but float past them, realizing that as the days pass, these memories will become fainter and fainter until they are replaced by happy ones. Also, as this happens, the knowledge that you are recovering brings its own joy and relief and helps you to forget past suffering. To sit peacefully and talk to a friend will at first be a wonder and a delight. Gradually you accept it as part of normal living, and that is how it should be.

"Oh, Not Again!"

Sometimes, perhaps weeks, even months after returning home and when you have forgotten the sharp edges of your illness, some reminder of it may catch you unaware and momentarily bring back some of the old sensations. At first you may be frightened and think, "Oh, not again!" But you will then remember how you cured yourself in the past and will realize that you could do the same again if need be, and your fears will calm and you will think, "Why bother to let it all start again?" And you don't bother. You float past the upsetting reminder.

Never Lost in That Maze Again

Your inner core of confidence is there, firm as a rock against any destructive suggestion. This is your security against all further nervous illness. You understand and therefore are unafraid. You know the way in, but you also know the way out. YOU WILL NEVER BE LOST IN THAT MAZE AGAIN. YOU HAVE BEEN RESCUED FROM BEWILDERMENT.

So:

Return home with confidence.
Recognize the difference between memory and reality.
Do not be bluffed by memory.

Facing Again What Made You Ill

It is very encouraging if, when you are about to return home after recovering from nervous illness, your family says, "Everything's been changed at home. We understand what made you ill. You won't have to face that again." You can now sail home with all flags flying. But more usually the family says, "You've been away for months. You should be cured by now. So the sooner you can come home, the better." No mention of changing anything.

You Can Think
Without too Much Feeling

Removal from the source of trouble allows time for emotions to calm, so that when you think of your problems your revulsive reactions are probably less severe. You have had time to acquire a certain insulation which helps you to "rise above the situation." To put it another way, your sensitized adrenalin-releasing nerves, removed from the source of constant irritation, have had time to recover and no longer shoot off exaggerated responses at the mere thought of your trouble. You can think without too much feeling.

Take Home a Definite Plan of Action

So far so good. But simply to return calmer and hoping for the best is not good enough. You are too vulnerable. Underneath your newly acquired calmness you are wondering how long your new suit of armor will last without cracking. To feel more secure you must take home a definite plan of action. You must have an acceptable way of looking at your problem before you return.

If your past suffering was severe enough to cause a nervous illness and if, on returning home, you must face the same source of suffering, it is obvious that you must have very good reasons for returning to it. The natural inclination is to run in the opposite direction.

If you are going home simply because there is nowhere else to go, possibly because you have no money and no training to earn money, and no desire to take a job that requires no special training—even though this may mean living in peace away from home—then admit that you are not a poor, persecuted human whose head fate insists on putting on the block, but a very usual sort of person who insists on putting his own head on the block. Stop regarding yourself as a martyr. With the martyr element honestly eliminated, the situation at home will seem less intolerable. Somehow, what comes will not seem so bad when you admit that returning to it is really your own choice.

TAKE YOUR HEAD OFF THE BLOCK

For example, if you are the mother of children, returning to a husband who spends his evenings away from home and who comes home the worse for drink, then you are obviously going back because you have decided that he is not such a bad father when sober and that it is better for the children to have a home with him in it than without him. So, instead of working yourself up while he is out at night, put his meal in the oven and find another interest. You have elected to make a home for the children, so make it a home, not a battleground. It is amazing how, once you change your way of looking at a situation, the situation itself may change.

So:

Understand why you are returning home.
Keep this firmly in mind.
Take your head off the block and make the most of the situation.

22

Apprehension

THE SHADOW OF THE SHADOW

Although the person recovering from nervous illness is no longer as afraid as he was, he may be unable to lose a feeling of apprehension. This perplexes him. He thinks, "Why should I still have this vague feeling of anxiety, as if something terrible is about to happen? I have nothing to worry about now, why should I feel like this?"

This feeling is most likely to come when he first wakes in the morning, before he has time to review the now more cheerful aspects of the situation and re-orient himself. It is an emotional habit, brought on by the months or years of true anxiety. It has been called the "shadow of the shadow."

LISTENING FOR THE KEY IN THE DOOR

Most of us have experienced this feeling. It is common in middle age when many become lost in sorrow. The health we accepted as our right, the body we have not had to worry about previously may give us a nasty shock and we could find ourselves faced with one or more spells in the hospital. Also, domestic troubles are most likely to come at this time. Parents must be nursed through long illnesses and lost in death. The growing family is at an age when they may cause grave concern, and many nights and early-morning hours may be spent listening for the key in the door before sleep will come. Troubles may follow in such rapid succession that, even when absent, we feel as if they are hovering in the background waiting to return.

Time and acceptance alone can dispel this. However, they may take so long to do their work that the sufferer may seek a doctor's help.

The patient often describes herself (it is usually a woman) as feeling more "flattened" than actually depressed or unhappy. She is easily discouraged. She thinks, "Wouldn't it be nice to see Alice?" but when she considers bathing and dressing she doesn't want to go. If Alice could materialize and say a few words, she would quite enjoy it, but to dress and catch a bus? No, that is too much! Planning any pleasure ahead is a burden.

These people sometimes come to the doctor almost in tears. They think they have a real problem. How are they to become themselves again? Are they going mad? Or (hopefully) is this the "change"?

Most people are greatly relieved to hear that they are no different from many others who have passed through this period of life. They are especially comforted to understand that their trouble is an emotional habit, is not mental, and that they can be cured.

THE EFFORT TO SEE ALICE

The cure is the same for you if, on recovering from nervous illness, you are left with a background of anxiety you cannot understand. You must lose the habit of carrying anxiety around. First, *make the effort to go and see Alice.* A habit must be broken, a shadow's shadow lost, and the quickest way to do this is to replace it with other memories, other feelings. It is surprising how close to the surface normal feelings lie when you once make the effort to rid yourself of the shadow of the shadow. You might start out to see Alice feeling as if you couldn't care less if the bus were to go on to Timbuktu, but after Alice has talked about herself for half an hour and you have talked about yourself for an hour, it is surprising how much better you feel. On the return bus journey you may even find yourself moving up amicably to make room for someone.

It is not easy to find the same lift by staying at home and merely lecturing to yourself while waiting for time to pass. It is a great help to get away from the house, where the shadow feels too much at home. It is essential to meet other people. Many middle-aged housewives go to work temporarily to help lose this feeling, and they are so much better for the daily change of scene that that which began as temporary occupation becomes permanent.

You can also help to change the daily pattern of your feelings by spoiling yourself a little each day. For example, a housewife once wrote to a journal describing how she overcame such a condition by some small, daily self-indulgence. When she saw violets on the flower stall, instead of thinking, as was her previous habit, "Such a price to pay for violets! What an extravagance!" she bought them and made a point of enjoying them throughout the day, stopping to smell and admire them. She was changing the pattern of her emotions by purposely introducing happy moments.

Indulge yourself in this way, so that you will grow used to the feeling of happiness again and it will gradually replace anxiety. Make the effort to help the shadow of the shadow to pass, and don't forget the violets.

23

Three Good Friends: Occupation, Courage, Religion

By now you will appreciate that what is known as nervous illness is no more than extreme emotional and mental fatigue usually begun and maintained by fear. Most of us experience, to some degree, suffering of this kind during the normal course of our lives, so that we could say that nervous illness is but an accentuation of such normal experience. There is no monster waiting to devour us; no precipice over which we will fall "if we don't look out"; no special point beyond which recovery is particularly difficult. *Anywhere, at any time during the illness, if we lose our fears, we can step out of it;* perhaps not immediately, but in a surprisingly short time.

You may feel that fate is ready to push you back at every opportunity during your recovery, but you can be cheered by the thought that, whatever fate may do, three good friends will never fail you—occupation, courage, and religion.

OCCUPATION

As I have so often stressed before, idleness, to a nervously ill person, can be a torture, each moment an eternity, and the strain almost unbearable. The exhausted mind races agitatedly and yet watches each second pass. No amount of self-chastisement can stop it. It seems almost beyond the powers of the sufferer to free himself from this situation, unless he has some crutch on which to rest his tired mind. Occupation in the company of others is his best crutch. But it is essential that he is not still bewildered by his problems and is not throwing himself into occupation as a way of fighting them. This leads to greater exhaustion and more bewilderment.

This person must first *find some solution or compromise for his problem, seeking advice where necessary; he must be prepared to cease fighting and float forward to recovery, accepting all the tricks his nerves play on him while attempting to lose himself in occupation.*

While occupied, one can, as it were, divide one's mind into two parts, the part that suffers and a new part that accepts and floats on. In spite of this new approach, the part that suffers will probably continue to suffer to some extent, with trouble hovering in the background, *but in the background.* It is now that occupation is such a blessing. It claims attention and acts like a splint for the tired mind, replacing painful by impersonal thought, so that the suffering gradually recedes. I repeat *that this happens only when the emotional pattern is acceptance and looking forward to future healing without resistance, resentment, fighting, and fear.*

THE MIDDLE-AGED MAN

Unfortunately many nervously ill people are middle-aged, and it is not easy to find suitable occupation for them. Middle-aged men are easier to help than women. A man can often continue at his work, which usually provides a daily change of scene and company.

One middle-aged man had been representing his firm abroad on an undertaking that involved mental strain, competition, arduous travel against time, and little sleep. He became exhausted when he needed his wits about him and he panicked at the thought of failure. He completed his work and returned home, but by this time was well advanced in a nervous "collapse," which he suffered for two years. He was given various treatments without lasting benefit, and when I saw him he was desperate. He explained that he was so ill that each thought was a burden. This was particularly upsetting because his work as an engineer entailed intricate thinking. He had tried many times to return to work, but each time had given up in despair and had returned home a worse wreck than ever. Nobody, said he, could have fought harder. I showed him where he had made his mistakes and advised what to do. He said, "What you say seems too simple. But I will try your way."

WHAT A MAGNIFICENT MECHANISM!

As he was physically exhausted, I prescribed light occupation at home for a few weeks, reconditioning an old car. At the end of this time he was improved, but still afraid to return to work and risk failure. Once again I pointed out his mistakes in the past. I explained that his brain was not damaged, as he thought; that it was as capable as ever of complicated reckoning, but could work only at a slow pace. I also showed him how previously, when he had begun to calculate, he had first put up a barrier of fear and lack of confidence. How could he expect a fatigued and therefore highly suggestible mind to overcome this and work satisfactorily? His brain was so exhausted by despairing thought, small wonder that it could only plod along. What a magnificent mechanism to function at all in these circumstances!

THINK AS SLOWLY AS A TIRED MIND ALLOWS

I pointed out that he must be prepared to attempt his engineering problems many times before he could solve them. He must accept that at the moment there may be some, perhaps many, he could not solve. *On no account must he make an issue of solving them, trying to prove to himself he could do it.* He must relax to the best of his ability, breathe quietly and calmly, and be prepared to think as slowly as his tired mind allowed him. In the circumstances how could it think quickly?

Also, he must not worry about how foolish he might look to others. What matter they? Who knows, the day might come when one of them would knock on his door for help.

Again and again I explained that the quality of thought was not changed, only its rate slowed by fatigue born of tension and fear.

This man recovered after some months of doing as advised. It was not easy, but no worthwhile success is easy. He is now a leading executive of his firm and a much more soundly integrated person than before his illness. What is just as important, he is no longer vulnerable. If his nerves start to play their old tricks, *he relaxes and accepts them,* does not attempt to fight them. Relaxation and acceptance give little encouragement to nervous illness.

This man was fortunate in that he had favorable conditions in which to recover. His position was waiting for him and he could return to it as gradually as he wished.

An Understanding Wife Stood Beside Him

Also, an understanding wife stood beside him, even though at times she was hurt, frightened, and bewildered. The doctor can do much if he takes the time to explain nervous illness to such a wife.

The situation between husband and wife can become complicated. The husband, if he is the sufferer, unable to make up his own exhausted mind, may turn to his wife for guidance over small details. Then, feeling himself a weakling for so doing, he will act against her advice in some pathetic effort to reassert his manhood and re-establish his dignity in his own and his wife's eyes. It is not surprising that some wives become desperate.

MIDDLE-AGED HOUSEWIFE

A man, with occupation normally away from home, usually keeps his troubles more in perspective and recovers from nervous illness more quickly than a housewife who is left to make beds, sweep floors, and wash up, with only tradesmen or children to talk to. There is little about the work to distract her. She does it automatically and in a place where she is constantly reminded of her suffering. It was while washing up that she had her first attack of palpitations, so the sink now holds new fears for her. Also the family of most middle-aged women have left home, so that the housework is lighter, is finished by midday or earlier, and the woman is left with the long, weary afternoon hours to fill in. She cannot always spend time with her neighbors, however co-operative they may be.

"TALK TO MY LITTLE DOG"

A lonely sick housewife described in writing how she felt after the family had left for the day. Her words are reproduced here without alteration. She wrote, "A feeling sweeps over me. I get hot, my face burns, my throat keeps swallowing, my lips get dry and tremble. I cry and feel as though I am going to smother. My tummy is churning. I feel I don't want to be alone. I close my hands, they are tense. My neck muscles get tense. My legs get wobbly. My head feels tight and feels as though it is going to lift. I now want to clench my hands. I have sat down at the veranda table. This is something I have been unable to do before. Before when I felt this turn coming on, my first impulse was to go outside and walk about. I now feel a little better. My husband has gone. I felt awful when he drove away. I am going to try and be sensible and go inside and wash up and talk to my little dog."

"Tomorrow They Are Going Early!"

The next day she wrote, "I woke up thinking I should go with my husband. But he could not take me. Later the feeling of being alone swept over me. Tomorrow they are going early. This seems to be a big problem. I get a feeling as though I am smothering and the walls are closing around me. I still feel tense and will try and do some housework. I will have to wait all day now until they come home. This seems a big problem."

Surely it is obvious that this woman should never have been left alone trying to cope with those long hours before her.

If such a person is unable to leave home temporarily, it is most helpful for the doctor to visit the home and see the conditions under which the patient is trying to recover. I had advised the woman just described to sit on her porch rather than stay indoors, and she had conscientiously done so, with little good result. I had not known until I saw it that the porch was enclosed by a high wooden partition and that, when seated, she could not see out. I requested that the partition be lowered immediately, but I first removed this woman elsewhere.

For the housewife, I try to find creative occupation different from housework and yet not demanding too much concentration. It is sometimes difficult to convince a husband that it is better for his wife to attend a class in the making of artificial flowers than to be home cooking his dinner. "If she can fiddle with flowers, why can't she cook supper?"

If you are a nervously sick housewife, do not feel guilty if you want to leave the dishes, make artificial flowers, breed dogs, or dig in the garden. Housework is rarely interesting to a woman with nervous illness, and since interest is the force that will help to lift you off the bed and out of illness, find it where you reasonably can.

A woman to whom I was recently called lay on a couch while being interviewed. She apologized for the state of the house, in particular for the state of the back veranda, saying that she had not the strength to work and that the veranda should have been painted months ago.

I suggested that she should start painting it the next day. She looked at me in amazement. How could she paint a house when she could hardly walk from one room to another? I could see her wondering what kind of doctor had been foisted on her.

I asked how long she had been on the couch and she answered, "Three months."

"Are you better for it?" I inquired.

She thought awhile and said, "No, I'm not. I guess that's why they've called you in."

I assured her I was not joking about the painting, and asked her skeptical husband to assemble the necessary implements by the next day. She could begin with scraping the paint from one of the window frames. This was not as strenuous as it sounded, because I had noticed that the paint was already peeling off in long strips.

THE EFFORT OF GETTING OFF THAT COUCH!

I also assured her that it was not important if at the first attempt she could scrape for only a few minutes. *It was the attempt that was important,* the effort of getting off that couch and facing a new task. I explained that she could not damage her body by making such effort, that indeed her muscles would regain their ability to function normally *only if she used them.* Muscles that have not been used for some time always complain when first used again. Their aching is only their peevish protest, not a measure of damage done by their re-use. In fact, in spite of such aching they will regain their normal strength much more quickly when used than when laid aside to rest.

CURED BY INTEREST

When I called a few days later she was gently scraping the window frame, in between sitting on a chair strategically placed nearby. A week later she was at the undercoat stage, and we had a brisk discussion about the color of the final coat. We settled for French gray walls and a Chinese red door. The thought of the red door acted like a magnet. She forgot her "poor weak legs" and almost ran to the garage to find the paint to show me. The next week our conversation was more about the painting than the illness. She was cured by interest in doing something refreshingly different. Confidence in her own strength was restored by using it.

I am not saying that this woman's tiredness was imaginary and that all she had to do was to pick up her bed and walk. The tiredness of nervous illness is real and may require some daily rest, but only a certain amount.

The sufferer may complain, and how often she does, that she is too exhausted to work. She is almost right, but only almost. Emotional stress may have reduced her to nothing more than skin and bone, but, however weak she may be, she is better out of bed and occupied somehow. The body will recover as the mind finds peace, and the mind is more likely to find peace when occupied than when brooding. An hour spent in bed in panic will exhaust more than light occupation will. Your body is ready to obey any reasonable demand, however exhausted you may think yourself, provided your interest is in what you are doing and not in watching your body work for fear you may "overdo it."

An American doctor worked so strenuously in Greece after World War I that when the last day of her appointment came and she was about to sail for home, she almost collapsed, saying she could not have worked another day. A few hours later she received a cable sending her immediately to work in South Russia. Now,

her one regret on going home had been that she had
not seen Russia. She became so interested in her new
appointment that she started working at full speed and
forgot to collapse. We are usually exhausted more in
spirit than in body. However, I emphasize that your
doctor must have examined you and diagnosed your
trouble as "only nerves."

FEAR OF "OVERDOING IT"

The patient is bound to overdo it occasionally, often
in the beginning. It is not unusual to find him in a
quandry trying to estimate how much work he should
attempt so as not to overtire himself. My advice is
always the same: while it is unwise to undertake tasks
that are obviously too strenuous, it is better to work and
risk overtiring yourself than to do nothing for fear of
it. But it is important that when you do overtire yourself, you do not lose confidence and waste additional
energy regretting and wondering "Why?" There will
probably be many such episodes before you are completely cured. If you accept the fatigue calmly, rest
and work again, you take two steps forward to each
step back.

ORGANIZED OCCUPATION

It is always difficult for a doctor to find occupation
for his patients. How much easier our work would be,
and how few patients would need shock treatment,
if there were places organized by the medical profes-
sion where people harassed by nerves could be kept
occupied and away from home. By such a place I do
not mean a hospital where the patient mixes with other
patients and the atmosphere is laden with talk of
nerves, their treatment and complications. I mean such
places as farms, schools, etc., that would be willing
to find bed and occupation for some of these people,
who would then be able to work and recover in normal
surroundings. Much of the good that comes from hos-

pital treatment for nerves is achieved mainly by removing the patient from familiar, distressful surroundings. Even to be away from the strain of being watched by an anxious family must be a relief.

I do not wish to decry the good work done by hospitals, but I do consider that a person with nervous illness who recovers in normal surroundings has a better chance of being more firmly integrated and more soundly rehabilitated than one who is treated in a hospital. The one in normal surroundings is actually being rehabilitated while being cured. Also, it is better for his morale and needs less explanation to inquisitive acquaintances.

It is a great help if such a person can, like the engineer described at the beginning of this section, continue at his usual work while awaiting cure. Occupation is there, already found, and he does not have the strain of meeting any embarrassing situation that may occur on returning to work after a prolonged absence with nervous illness. Also, he quickly loses any feeling of strangeness that his illness may have brought him. Fitting into a normal pattern helps him to feel more normal. However, it may be difficult for him to remain at his usual work because he may find it too much strain to keep to a schedule. People with nervous illness can do a great deal at their own pace, but if asked to work to a fixed time or keep an appointment punctually, they may feel incapacitated by the strain of anticipation.

THE STRAIN OF A SET APPOINTMENT

For example, the nervously ill mother of two small boys had progressed so well away from home that she was soon able to return each day to clean part of the house and help prepare the evening meal. When the school holidays arrived it became necessary for someone to be with the boys each morning when the father left for work. He naturally expected the mother to be there. After all, she was well enough to do nearly everything else by now, why not come at eight o'clock each morning instead of drifting in at any hour of the day? What difference? His wife soon taught him the difference. She went to pieces at the mere suggestion. She simply could not take the strain of a set appointment. She explained that to know she must be with the boys by eight in the morning was enough to banish sleep the night before. She felt she could not tolerate the strain of waiting for the hours to pass until morning came and wanted to relieve it by rushing home immediately.

THE FAMILY MAY LISTEN WITH DISAPPROVAL

I try to impress on the family the importance of keeping such strain from the patient during the early weeks of convalescence. Sometimes they listen with disapproval. They think that if Mother was obliged to do such and such she would be much better for it. If Mother did such and such she would probably be better for it, but not if she was obliged to.

Finding suitable occupation is a problem that must be met and solved with each patient. I can but emphasize the absolute necessity for it. If further proof is needed, one has but to compare the patient on Friday with the same person on Monday after an idle weekend. So often there is deterioration. "Sundays nearly kill me," say so many.

There is a special type of isolation treatment, where the "nerve" patient is put to bed in a hospital and isolated from outside contacts. This may work for some, but the risk is great. It is too much strain for a tired mind to be thrown on its own resources for hours, days, on end. I repeat again and again, be occupied. *Let occupation be your crutch.*

Do not misunderstand and feverishly seek occupation, fearing to be idle. Moderation in all things, even here. Occupation can be interspersed with rest. But it is better to err on the side of too much activity than too much rest.

"If He Had Had Company for Just a Few More Days"

The company of others is just as important as occupation. Some years ago a young man described an illuminating experience he had had while recovering from nervous illness. He was staying with friends in the country, where he was obliged to be alone most of the day. One of the friends was unexpectedly home for two weeks, so that, for that short time, the sick man had continuous companionship. At the end of the fortnight he was much improved, and he described how desperate he felt when the time came to be alone again during the day. He said he knew that had he had company for just a few more days, the rest this would have given his tired mind would have been just enough to allow him to find the command over his thoughts he so desperately sought. As it was, he had the distressing experience of watching himself slip back and lose some of the ground gained, knowing there was little he could do but accept the situation philosophically and wait for more time to pass.

The Still, Pressing Solitude of the Country

This man should have had occupation with daily companionship and not a quiet country holiday. Quietness is often mistakenly prescribed for "nerves." It may be easier for some people to recover from nervous illness in the noisy distractions of the city rather than in the still, pressing solitude of the country.
So:

Let occupation be your crutch.
Accept all the tricks your nerves play on you while attempting to lose yourself in occupation.
Relax, accept the temporary slowness of your thought, and be prepared to think as slowly as your tired brain allows; time and peace will bring full recovery.

If you are a housewife, do not stay alone all day; find interest away from home.

Seek occupation in the company of others.

Remember, an hour spent in bed in panic will exhaust you more than light occupation will, so get off that bed.

COURAGE

Courage has the extraordinary quality of being there *if truly wanted*. If you want, earnestly enough, to be courageous, you will be. If you fail, re-examine yourself and you will find you have misled yourself. You only thought you wanted to be brave, you did not actually feel the urge. To be conscious of a real urge, you must feel it strongly within yourself, in the pit of your stomach, so that you can almost put your finger on the spot. In other words, this wanting must come well forward in your consciousness and not be tucked away, overlaid by wishy-washy wishing.

You must establish and cultivate this feeling until you make it part of yourself. There is nothing difficult or illusory about this. It is almost a trick, like the trick of floating. Lie still and close your eyes and think of something you want very much, something for which you have a deep yearning. It is here, where you feel this yearning, that you will also feel courage and confidence: always the pit of the stomach. In the beginning be satisfied if you feel only a yearning for courage. If you persevere, with practice it will become courage itself. But first make sure that you feel it. *Feel the yearning* in your stomach, *do not only think it* in your head.

It is unfortunate that our training does not help us to bring such positive inner feelings more easily to our assistance. When young we are taught what to do, think, and feel, until we react to the pattern laid down by our training. Our true selves, our real possibilities, we rarely uncover, and we can and usually do go from cradle to grave without knowing what we, the true you and I, honestly think, believe, or feel.

So do not be satisfied with the mere wish you may now feel to be brave and persevering. Give your desire so much concentration that you eventually make it a granitelike determination to succeed. If you take time to do this, your journey to recovery will be winged.

It is curious how this feeling of courage and confidence seems to be seated, not in our brain, but in our "middle." This is a good place to feel it—it adds strength to our "backbone."

"WHAT'S THE USE OF CRYING IN THE DARK?"

A doctor has a unique opportunity to see examples of great courage. After years of practice, the average doctor emerges with respect and love for his fellows. They have their faults, but their courage makes these faults easy to forgive. An old patient of mine, a woman of eighty-two, suffered one of the most trying illnesses known. One night, after she had had a particularly grueling day, I went into her room expecting her to be in despair. Instead, I found her listening to the radio and reading from a book of short stories.

I said in amazement, "I did not expect to find you cheerfully reading like this."

She looked at me quizzically and answered, "What's the use of crying in the dark?" This book is dedicated to the memory of that patient.

To get such courage *you must want it*. When you finally have it, it will stand between you and all future adversity, between you and failure. Find it, as I have suggested, and if you lose it, search again. And there will be no more crying in the dark.

RELIGION

The religious have faith in God to help them. But those who are not religious find little comfort in being told to put their trust in God and pray for help. They would of course recover if they did, but even those with such faith sometimes have to be shown the actual steps to recovery. Sometimes religious people think they are being tried by God or tempted by the devil, and they fight all the harder to justify themselves before the one and master the other, only exhausting themselves in the effort.

The person who bears his suffering with patience (letting more time pass), and resignation (acceptance) and faith that God will cure him has found the way to recovery, but many get lost on the way and forget how to apply their faith.

Again, some nervously sick religious people complain of being unable to contact their religion, like the mother who could not contact her family. This is an added worry, especially when they find no solace in prayer. When they understand that they feel this way simply because their emotions are exhausted, they are greatly relieved.

So to tell people to put their faith in God and let Him cure them works only for those who have such faith and know how to apply it. These are indeed blessed. The others must be shown the way.

24

Dos And Don'ts

---

1. Do not run away from fear. Analyze it and see it as no more than a physical feeling. Do not be bluffed by a physical feeling.
2. Accept all the strange sensations connected with your illness. Do not fight them. Float past them. Recognize that they are temporary.
3. Let there be no self-pity.
4. Settle your problem as quickly as you can, if not with action, then by glimpsing and accepting a new point of view.
5. Waste no time on "What might have been" and "If only . . ."
6. Face sorrow and know that time will bring relief.
7. Be occupied. Do not lie in bed brooding. Be occupied calmly, not feverishly trying to forget yourself.
8. Remember that the strength in a muscle may depend on the confidence with which it is used.
9. Accept your obsessions and be prepared to live with them temporarily. Do not fight them by trying to push them away. Let time do that.
10. Remember, your recovery does not necessarily depend "entirely on you," as so many people are so ready to tell you. You may need help. Accept it willingly, without shame.
11. Do not measure your progress day by day. Don't count the months, years you have been ill and despair at the thought of them. Once you are on

the right road to recovery, recovery is inevitable, however protracted your illness may have been.

12. Remember, withdrawal is your jailer. Recovery lies on the other side of panic. Recovery lies in the places you fear.

13. Do not be discouraged if you cannot make decisions while you are ill. When you are well, decisions will be more easily made.

14. Never accept total defeat. It is never too late to give yourself another chance.

15. Practice, don't test.

16. *Face. Accept. Float. Let time pass.*

If you do this, you will recover.

25

Taking the First Steps

If you have read as far as this chapter and understand what I have been teaching but are afraid to take the first steps, it is usually because of one or all of the following reasons:

1. You have been ill so long you doubt your ability to recover. You think you are chronically sick.
2. You have no confidence in yourself to do what I ask. You have let yourself down so often in the past that you haven't the heart to trust yourself again.
3. You understand what I advise but it seems as if your body won't do it for you. It shoots off such lightning thrusts that you seem to crumble before them.
4. You feel so emotionally, mentally, and physically exhausted that you think you have not the strength to take that first step. That first step seems like a step to the land of Never Never.

Let us examine these reasons in detail.

1. You think you have been ill too long to recover. First understand that there is no "thing" doing this to you. Your reactions, although they may seem devastating, are superficial and are merely your body's response to the way you think. Change the way you think and your reactions will change. The healing power is within you just as strongly as within anyone

else, *however long you may have suffered*. Your body is not resentful because you have handled it wrongly all these months, years. It bears no grudge. It is ready to start the processes of recovery as soon as you step out of its way. I have had people come to me who have been ill for the greater part of their life, and yet they have recovered when shown what to do. Long illness means only that the habit of being ill is firmly entrenched, memory discouraging, despair so readily at hand. All this can be changed by your attitude.

There is no such thing as a chronic state of nervous illness that cannot be cured once you understand what is needed from you and once you are determined to carry out instructions.

2. You have no confidence in yourself. You don't trust yourself.

It doesn't matter if you don't trust yourself. I'm not asking you to trust yourself. I am asking you to understand and trust the advice I have given you. I assure you it works. But I am not asking for blind trust. I have given you explanation for every important symptom, almost every strange experience. I want your understanding, not your blind faith. If you understand, as I said at the beginning of the book, it doesn't matter how big a coward you may think yourself at this moment, the method will still work if you follow it. You do not have to cure yourself. Your body will cure itself, if you practice spotting *second* fear and sending it packing.

3. You understand, but it is as if your body will not obey you.

If you are like this, you must be very sensitized, so you will have to accept much *first* fear for a while. You probably think that when panic strikes, you cannot think at all and simply cannot practice going through it with acceptance. But this is not so. You can think well enough to think, "Let me out of here, quickly!" or, "This is more than I can stand!" However severe the panic, if you watch yourself at the moment when panic flashes most acutely, you will find that you can still think, even if the wrong thoughts! I want you to practice not shrinking from that flash, wherever it may seem to carry you. If you fear it will carry you into oblivion, *then be prepared to go into oblivion. But go willingly.* You won't go into oblivion. You are being bluffed by intense feeling and imagination.

What I teach is not easy, but it is all possible. It is rather like learning to ride a bicycle. There is a lot of wibbling and wobbling and falling off, but unless you pick yourself up when you fall and practice again, you will never ride that bicycle. So do not be dismayed by failure at practicing acceptance. Practice, practice, practice until panic comes to mean so little that *it eventually turns itself off before it starts.*

4. You think you have not the strength to take the first step.

Remember that the weakness that comes with nervous illness is not true, muscular, organic weakness, so don't let it bluff you. "Nerves" can so easily bluff the nervously ill, because the weakness they bring can be so debilitating and seem so real. However weak and ill you may feel, your muscles will grow stronger only as you begin to use them. I remind you that I am assuming that you have your doctor's assurance that you are suffering "only from nerves."

Your doctor may suggest rest and sedation for a short while. Be guided by him. But be off that bed as soon as he gives the word. However hesitatingly you may take those first steps, *take them.* They are the first steps to recovery.

26

Advice to the Family

The family of the person with nervous illness often accuses him of being a complete egoist. Many mothers complain, "If I could be more sure my daughter were ill, and not just selfish, it would be much easier to put up with her. But, Doctor, she is completely wrapped up in herself. It doesn't seem to matter to her that she has exhausted me and brought us all to the verge of breakdown with her!"

Perhaps you feel this way about some member of your family. If you have found time to read this book, a new understanding should help you to forgive such apparent egoism.

An author or composer in the throes of creating is so engrossed in his work that he may hardly be aware of what goes on around him and may so take for granted the comfort and peace provided by a pair of hands in the background that he fails to notice how lonely, neglected, and even fed up the owner of the hands may be. A perfect egoist, but simply because of such demanding absorption elsewhere.

A TYPE OF EGOIST

A seriously ill person is a somewhat similar type of egoist. In the beginning, his illness was probably caused by some disturbing problem, the continuous contemplation of which exhausted him and brought such alarming bodily sensations that other people's troubles seemed non-existent in comparison. Had he let himself become too aware of his family's concern about him, the added strain would have seemed unbearable. So, in self-defence, he shied away from such awareness, even to the point of appearing callous and egoistical. In addition, his needs are usually accompanied by such a strained urge for immediate appeasement that in his agitation to get relief he is quite capable of ruthlessly brushing aside the needs of others.

If you can see this relative as a sick person who, when well, will be no more egoistical than the rest of us, it will help you to tolerate and aid now. Of course, if he was always selfish and his present state is but an accentuation of this, it is more difficult to tolerate him. Even here, show compassion for someone whose suffering is real and desperate and do not begrudge your sympathy or help.

SYMPATHY

The family is often warned against sympathizing with the sufferer and unfortunately may take the warning too literally and be too hard on him. Do not be afraid to sympathize and show that you are trying to understand. Sympathy and understanding can comfort and encourage a wracked spirit and relieve tension. However, do not encourage self-pity. Mix sympathy with a reminder that his problems are out of proportion and that as he improves they will not seem so insuperable. Above all, help to find, as soon as possible, a solution or compromise for those problems, and so save him from exhausting cogitation. It is the everlasting worrying, thinking, and feeling intensely that is exhausting him.

If the problems cannot be solved, at least help him to find a less distressing way of looking at them and living with them. You may both have to discuss a new point of view many times before he can see it and hold it as his own. Try not to lose patience, however often he returns for such discussion.

A Program of Light Work

Make sure that the sufferer is kept occupied. By this I do not mean that you must direct him back to work whenever you see him idle. I mean have a program of light work organized, so that it is ready for him. He may work only fitfully in the beginning, for his staying power will be limited. This is not important. But it is important that the occupation is there and that he is not left continually idle.

If your relative is a housewife, on no account must she be left alone all day. All the sympathy and help in the world given in the evening will not compensate for a day spent in the house with no company other than her own thoughts. I must repeat and insist on the importance of occupation in the company of others, particularly for a housewife, and ask you not to procrastinate in finding it.

Many families are willing to pay the expenses of a relative's illness but fail when it comes to finding occupation for her. This is frustrating because the doctor can bring the patient only to a certain point of recovery, where occupation is essential to complete it. I explain this to every family and yet at each visit so many find some fresh excuse for not having done as requested. Please make every effort to find satisfactory occupation for your relative.

Auntie Maud Who Lives
Three Hundred Miles Away

It is a great temptation when casting around desperately for a suitable sanctuary for your sick relative to think of Auntie Maud who lives three hundred miles away at Bargo Bargo in a dear little cottage on the side of a hill overlooking a river that leads, after half an hour's walk, to another dear little cottage on the other side of the hill. It is a great temptation to think that the peace and quiet, the lovely fresh air and the fresh cream will just fix Mary. Unfortunately that's just what they might do, but not the way you want Mary fixed. Mary may need company, change, distraction, constant diversion, and not the lonely sound of the boobook owl, however fresh the air around it. To sit for an hour and sip a soda at a busy store and watch people come and go will help many people with nervous illness much more than the fresh air in the lonely silence of the mountains. Depressed spirits depend so much on outside environment to help them. They have no inner source of joy to support them. They are like a weathercock that must turn this way and that with every changing breath of wind. In a sad, lonely atmosphere the spirit can sink to a depth of despair understood only by those who have experienced it. So, if your sick relative has chosen to go to the country but writes imploring to come home after having been there but a short time, bring her home without complaining.

MOLEHILLS THAT CAN BE MOUNTAINS

If your relative has a particular problem that you can solve, however trivial it may seem to you, solve it. For example, a nervously sick woman had two prize dogs about whom she was worried. Her husband promised to board them with a veterinary surgeon while she was away. When the time came to do this, he could not bring himself to spend so much money on two dogs, especially as it was needed urgently elsewhere. So, thinking he was acting wisely, he did not keep his promise. The wife, who was progressing well, as soon as she heard that the dogs were still at home, worried so much that the results of three weeks' psychotherapy were endangered. I tried to show the husband that, of all the money he was spending at the moment, that on the dogs was perhaps the best spent, wasted though it might seem to him.

I have described this incident because you may have a similar problem from time to time and may wonder why you should "give in" to your relative. Do not regard it as giving in, but as saving mental and emotional suffering when emotions are so exaggerated and vulnerable. What may seem a molehill to you is a mountain to the sufferer. However, I do not mean that you must placate this relative at every turn. If you use common sense mixed with gentle firmness, understanding, and sympathy, you will make few mistakes.

"FIGHT IT!" "PULL YOURSELF TOGETHER!"

Never tell your relative to "fight it." Tell him *not to fight it, to accept it;* to practice masterly inactivity and float past troublesome issues that cannot be resolved; to float past fear of the bodily sensations of his illness. He must float, not fight. This is the way!

Also, should you advise your relative to pull himself together, remember that you are talking to a sick person so affected by illness that to pull himself together would be literally to cure himself. You are, in reality, saying to him, "For goodness' sake, cure yourself, quickly and now!" I know of no advice more depressing to such a sick person than being told to pull himself together, because part of nervous illness is trying to find a way through bewilderment to do just that. So should you use this phrase, at least appreciate what you demand and be prepared to show your relative how to do it. He doesn't know. Do you?

Do not think that by saying, "Stop all this nonsense and go back to work!" you have shown him the way. Try to understand that to find the way to stop all "this nonsense" is his biggest problem. So much of the nonsense has become conditioned reflex action, and who has ever succeeded in quickly stopping that?

It is true that sometimes going back to work is enough to cure nervous illness. It does this by helping to take the sick person's mind temporarily off his problems long enough to refresh it so that he can face the problems with less emotional reaction. Also the normal atmosphere of his daily work highlights the unreality of his illness and gives him encouraging flashes of normality.

However, taking problems and fears back to work is often of no avail, and the patient may be severely set back by the added indignity of having once more to leave work and return home ill. He may have made, in his opinion, a "fool of himself." It is safe for the sufferer to return to work only when he has a program of recovery planned such as is outlined in this book. With a plan to support and guide him, he runs little risk of failure. So, I repeat, when you say, "Stop all this nonsense and go back to work," be sure you first show your relative how to stop the nonsense. I hope your compassion and interest have been aroused enough to prompt you to read this book and learn how to help him.

27

A Husband's Attitude to His Wife's Nervous Illness

I had just spent an hour with a sick woman. It was essential that I speak to her husband, and I found him polishing his car in the driveway. He continued polishing as I spoke and did not raise his eyes. After I had given a full explanation of his wife's condition and asked for his co-operation, he blurted out, "Mashed potato! Always mashed potato! Why not chipped potatoes?"

I explained as patiently as I could that his wife could not cope with three small children and chipped potatoes at the same time.

He was not convinced. "How much longer will she be like this?"

If she'd stop swallowing all those pills and pull up her socks, she'd be all right. He knew plenty of women with more children than his wife, and they weren't like this. This was stupid. This wasn't the girl he married. How soon would she be the girl he married?

This man did not mean to be cruel to his wife. He simply did not understand. Nervous illness is bewildering. Doctors disagree about cause and treatment so it is small wonder that husbands are perplexed. In the beginning this man sympathized with his wife, but when the illness dragged on, while the wife looked well enough, talked sensibly enough, he found it more and more difficult to remain patient. It seemed so silly to him that a woman of her age should be afraid to go shopping alone. He would look at her in amazement, unable to understand how his wife, the woman who took the "big operation" without a murmur, could now be afraid to go out without him. To mention going to the movies was enough to send her into a panic. When he asked "Why?" she would answer only, "I'm too frightened!" This was no explanation from a grown woman!

It was difficult for her to explain to a man without "a nerve in his body" how, while she waited in line at the shop, the tension would mount until it seemed unbearable and she would feel urged to run outside before she fainted, "collapsed," or "something terrible" happened. Small wonder the husband was confused when she returned without the food she had gone to buy. Surely it is not hard to understand why this man went on polishing his car, truculently demanding chipped potatoes. To him, home-cooked chips meant normal living. No wonder he wanted her to stop all the nonsense.

Alas! No one wanted this more than she, but finding a way to stop the nonsense meant finding her way to recovery, and until recently this had seemed beyond her.

It is not easy for a doctor to tell a man, harassed by an emotionally distressed wife, disturbed children, household bills, that his wife's quick recovery depends so much on his continued patience and that he must try to understand even when understanding seems so hard, so that he will add as little extra tension as possible to his wife's suffering.

A wife will say, "When I try to explain to my husband, Doctor, I can see by the look on his face that he thinks I'm crazy or something. It's not his fault. But I wish he wouldn't go to pieces so quickly when he sees me like this. I wish he wouldn't think he's helping me by trying to force me to do things. It's when he does this that the tension mounts, and that's what frightens me so much, Doctor."

A Husband Needs Encouragement

A husband's co-operation is so important that a doctor should explain as fully to him as to his wife what is happening and how she can be cured. A husband needs explanation, encouragement, and support, so that his criticism can be turned into constructive help. The added tension of being watched by a pair of critical eyes helps to keep a wife in a cycle of tension-worry-tension.

His Cross As Well As Hers

The husband has but to go off in a huff in the morning to throw his wife into despair for the day. He may forget about it until he reaches for his hat when his work is over, but she has been "with it" since he left. And you may be sure that, in his desperate state (and his is a desperate state) he delivered a few telling broadsides before leaving, especially that final thrust, as he closed the door, about the cross he bears. The woman, left alone with perhaps only children for company, or with no company at all, now has not only her cross to carry, but his as well.

Back on the Same Old Razzle-Dazzle

Of course she tries to talk sense to herself. Part of her trouble is arguing with herself and getting nowhere. One minute she decides to stop all this nonsense once and for all, to let none of it get her down; but the next she's at it again, back on the same old razzle-dazzle, back with, "Oh, my goodness" and "What if . . . ?"

The entire day is a battlefield strewn with good resolves and as many failures. No wonder she is confused and afraid of what is happening to her. She asks why everything should seem so impossible. If only her husband could understand how trapped she feels, how desperately she wants to be her old self again. If only he could understand that his inability to stay the course with his wife, his pressing urgency for her to recover, his tendency to belittle her illness are some of the main reasons for her delayed recovery.

LONG-PLAYING RECORDS

It is often difficult, even impossible, to persuade a husband to read this book. Here my long-playing records have a special mission. Many reluctant husbands find themselves listening despite themselves. Even disapproving relatives will listen out of curiosity to LP recordings, and it can be gratifying to the sufferer to hear them say later, "Now, I understand at last." *

ALL CHILDREN, FOOD, CHORES

Some aspects of housekeeping can hardly be called interesting, especially preparing food for children and trying to force it down reluctant throats or scraping it off the floor after losing the battle. The average mother puts up with this when well, because she mixes it with happier experiences. When nervously ill nothing may interest her. Life becomes all children, food, chores, and this adds to her confusion because *it used not to worry her like this.*

In nervous illness emotions are so grossly exaggerated that mild dislikes may become revulsions, and it may seem impossible for the mother to change them back into mild dislikes so that she can tolerate them again.

"POOR GEORGE! I DON'T KNOW HOW YOU HAVE PUT UP WITH IT FOR SO LONG!"

Some husbands withdraw from the situation. They've "had it" and find refuge away from home. Friends may not help. "Poor George! I don't know

---

*Dr. Weekes' album of two recordings on nervous illness is available from Galahad Productions, P.O. Box 4996, Washington, D.C. 20008. The price is $18.00.

how you have put up with it so long!" may be handed to George with a friendly drink, and if George hadn't already wondered himself, he certainly does now.

THE END OF HER TETHER

It is difficult to convince a man how much his wife's recovery may depend on him. It is a difficult task to say to a man, almost as exhausted as his wife, "However upset you are, however strained your patience, your nerves, you must try to be patient a little longer. If you are at the end of your tether, what about her? She saw the end of her tether months ago and she is still trying. Don't make your wife feel that everything depends on her quick recovery. That is too much for a sick woman to bear."

If a husband takes the trouble to try to understand and help, his reward will be the grateful, deep love of a wife who will never forget his strength, kindness, and dependability in her illness. If he does not, despite the many excuses she will make for him, she will find it hard to forget that he failed her when she needed him most, and her illness may drag on unnecessarily.

28

Fear of Recurring Nervous Illness

If you have been nervously ill at some time in the past, you probably dread the thought of experiencing it again. Most people say, "I hope I never break down again." Very few have the confidence to say, "I *will* never break down again." I want you to be able to say, and know, that you will never break down again.

YOUR ONLY ENEMY IS FEAR

If you are afraid of future nervous illness, you probably avoid thinking about it and are content to bury thought of it at the back of your mind and hope for the best. *This is not good enough*. In this condition you are subconsciously tensed and therefore vulnerable. If asked what you fear, you would probably hesitate and then list a number of dreaded possibilities, each related to your unhappy experience. I want you to be able to look clearly into the future and know that *your only enemy is fear*. Fear alone makes you vulnerable. Without fear there could be no future illness. *It is as simple as that*. Nervous illness is only an expression of sustained fear; *no more than the exaggerated physical expression of fear,* and the fatigue and tension it brings.

So, first appreciate that *it is fear and fear alone that can disarm you*. You are not obliged to fight the thought of having another breakdown in order to avert it. You need not bury thought of it at the back of your mind. You are not obliged to watch lest you become overtired and so make yourself more vulnerable to breakdown. To be free from all possibility of it in the future, you have but to unmask fear, expose it, analyze it, understand it, and recognize what an all-important part it played in your last illness. Understand that *without fear your adrenalin-releasing nerves lack the stimulus to excite your organs to produce the sensations of breakdown.* You remain calm, and no one has ever had a breakdown while calm.

Scientists have devised tablets to tranquilize the action of the adrenalin-releasing nerves in the hope of preventing threatened illness. But you can produce your own tranquility, your own invulnerability, if you do not shy from the thought of future breakdown, but face it squarely and see what can be done now to prevent it later.

THERE WAS A SOLUTION, WASN'T THERE?

There is much you can do. First, analyze your previous illness and honestly try to find its cause. This may not be easy, because you may have to search well beyond the previously supposed cause. I have no doubt that you will find that fear was the real cause. Having done this, review your experience in the light of this discovery and consider how you could have solved your problems had you not succumbed to fear. There was a solution, wasn't there? While you consider thus, you may for the first time face your previous illness honestly and may feel surprising relief.

Now consider the future and ask yourself what you would do if threatened by a similar situation. Would you let fear play as big a part in it as you did before? I doubt it. Especially since you now recognize that *unafraid you would be invulnerable to breakdown.*

To be even surer of freeing yourself from the bondage of fear, practice further unmasking it, "debunking" it. The next time you feel a spasm of fear, instead of shying away from it and trying to forget it or to control and prevent its coming, as you have done in the past,

I want you to examine it as it sweeps through you and even to describe it to yourself, noting in detail its various component sensations, and refraining from adding *second* fear.

When you do this, you will find that the wave of fear strikes hardest when it first strikes, and that if you stand your ground and relax, *it quietens and disappears.* When you have learned to face fear this way, and see it as no more than a physical feeling, *you begin to lose your fear of fear.* You step outside a vicious circle. A spasm may come from time to time, but you learn to disregard it.

LET THE FIRST SHOCK PASS

Now let us see how your conquest of the physical feeling of fear can affect your chances of avoiding future nervous illness. If you were able to convince yourself that fear was the main reason for your previous illness (there will be no doubt of this if you are honest), you can surely understand that it did so by interfering with your power to think rationally. Can you see how, uninfluenced by fear, your ability to think and act would be so much more efficient? You would be able *to let the first shock pass* and then cope with the problem.

In the earlier part of this book I advised floating past fear. This is another way to express the advice just given in this chapter. By "floating" I mean letting the wave of fear break and sweep past you while you carry on in spite of it. When you can do this, you will retain your ability to think calmly, and calamity can never completely overwhelm you again. There can be no future breakdown.

I do not mean that whenever you feel a wave of fear approaching you must meet and analyze it. As you lose your fear of fear, these spasms will mean less and less and you will lose interest in them. If one comes more fiercely than usual you will accept it and not give it undue attention.

After you have practiced as suggested, you will

gradually understand and begin to feel the confidence
you need so much to help you face the future calmly.
Never forget that *without fear, you are invulnerable,
however often you may have been nervously ill in the
past.*

29

What Kind of Person Suffers from Nervous Illness?

Anybody is capable of experiencing a nervous illness, although some will break (that is, fall victim to fear) more readily than others. Anybody given enough strain, sorrow, or conflict is capable of exhausting himself, and if he makes the mistake of becoming afraid of, and trying to fight, the manifestations of his sensitized nerves, he can easily be caught in the circle of fear-fight-fear that leads to illness.

THE CHILD WHO WAITS TENSELY AT DUSK

People can be helped or hindered by their early training. A child who waits at dusk, tense and afraid, for a drunken father to come home will not have the same calm nervous system as a child brought up in a happy family with a mother who sees that it goes to bed early and has a good night's sleep. Also, the child who is kept on the *qui vive* by an excitable parent is more easily aroused to exaggerated nervous reaction when the occasion arises than a child who is kept calm. Hysterical excitement is not good for the young. Let them look forward to happy events with pleasure, but not with exaggerated excitement. A calm word from Mother can do much. For example, instead of saying to a child, "Only two more weeks to Christmas, isn't it exciting?" how much more soothing and sensible to say,

"You have two whole weeks before Santa Claus comes, so there is plenty of time to enjoy something else meanwhile."

MODERATION

At school we are taught history, mathematics, etc., but rarely how to practice moderation and self-discipline. This is left to our parents to teach us, many of whom do not understand the meaning of the words, let alone their practice. Moderation and self-discipline are the most important part of our defense mechanism. The mature person can be moderate in all things, can free himself from emotional dictation, and act after suitable deliberation. It is difficult to act uninfluenced by feeling. If any one of us has to brush aside unpleasant emotional reaction to think reasonably, he finds it difficult to pass that emotional barrier. We are so often afraid of unpleasant feelings. We suspect that they may become more unpleasant if we face them, so we try to extinguish them before they become established.

LET THE FIRST SHOCK PASS

Unpleasant feeling is particularly unwelcome if we have been allowed to grow up with our feelings meaning too much to us, because an indulgent parent has quickly substituted what we liked for what we did not like. If like this we usually want quick release from unpleasantness and rarely wait for our emotions to calm before acting.

If our education had included training to bear unpleasantness and to *let the first shock pass* until we could think more calmly, many an apparently unbearable situation would become manageable, and many a nervous illness avoided. So much nervous illness is, as I have stressed in this book, no more than emotional and mental exhaustion following prolonged possession by unhappy and fearful emotions. There is a proverb expressing this. It says, "Trouble is a tunnel through which we pass and not a brick wall against which we must break our head."

A certain amount of suffering is good for us, particularly when young. We should not be sheltered too much. The experience you gain from your present suffering could be your staff in the years to come.

Index

Afterword

This book has attained such success since it was first published in the United States that it is now (1989) hailed by many, including therapists, as the best book of its kind. For example, Dr. Roger Baker, lecturer at Aberdeen University, Scotland, and editor of Wiley's well-known psychiatric textbooks, in this years volume, *Panic, Disorders: Theory, Research and Therapy*, wrote: "This book presents probably the best known therapy for panic-anxiety: that of Claire Weekes." Earlier in the book he wrote: "Her work goes on to ensure that our treatments are receptive on a long-term basis."

Dr. Robert DuPont, Clinical Professor of Psychiatry, Georgetown University, Washington, D.C., addressing the Washington 1981 Conference of the Phobia Society of America, said: "The books of Claire Weekes have done more to help phobic sufferers worldwide than all other treatment programs combined."

During the years since publication this book has been summarised in the *Readers' Digest*, featured in *Time* Magazine, published in many foreign languages including Japanese and Afrikaans, and produced in Braille in Washington, D.C., and has been selected by the World Book Club.

It is so successful because it offers what so many people have long searched for in vain—a simple, clear, full explanation of why they look at others in the street, thinking, "What has happened to me? Why can't I be like them, be the person I used to be?" With bewilderment gone, fear soon goes too, and with it, nervous illness.

The treatment offered here is particularly important today because it is the prime challenger to the present vogue of dependence on long-term and even lifetime use of tablets to redress "chemical imbalance" in nervous illness. True, there are some comparatively rare nervous disorders that need such treatment, and it is also true that some nervously ill people, when treated with tablets (tranquilizers, anti-depressants) find great relief, but the relief is usually only temporary. For lasting relief one must find recovery not in tablets but in oneself, by making one's own effort.

Nervously ill persons who depend on tablets are like tightrope walkers trying to stay balanced. The teachings in this book cannot only catch them if they fall but also stop them from falling.

—Claire Weekes
December 1989
Sydney, Australia

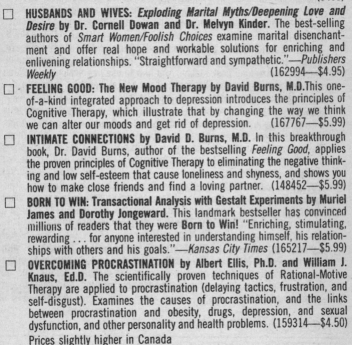